Praise for P

"*Pain Free* is based on a very sound understanding of human physiology. It shows how we can break the circuit of pain and naturally heal one of the most significant disabilities of our time."

—Deepak Chopra

"The ideas that Pete Egoscue brings to the world of nonoperative orthopedics are thoughtful, insightful, a bit controversial but undeniably USEFUL! In this book you will find very practical and quite often amazingly effective advice for dealing with joint pains and contractures. I have used many of Pete's thought-processes (and E-cises) in caring for my patients over the years; they work quite often, quite well. This is a short, easy-to-read, and actually pretty interesting book—buy it, read through—sooner or later you're going to need it!"

—Scott V. Haig, M.D., assistant clinical professor of orthopedic surgery, Columbia University, author of *Orthopedic Emergencies: A Radiographic Atlas*

"You don't have to be a professional athlete to find value in Pete's message. Whatever your walk in life, this book offers simple, sensible, and impactful advice. I've been blessed to have Pete and his team educate me throughout my career on how to get my body in the right positions for maximum performance. And this book is the cheat code. Quite simply, it's a game changer."

—Justin Tuck, former NFL All-Pro and Super Bowl Champion

"I have been a dedicated and consistent client and devotee of The Egoscue Method for over thirty years. It has not only changed my life but has been the foundation of my health and fitness. I arrived at Pete's clinic as a 25-year-old suffering from acute back pain related to a car crash. I was unable to play golf and had given up waterskiing, at 25! Within days, my posture changed, my gait changed, and I was completely out of pain. The Egoscue Method has enabled me to continue to play golf, water ski, and snow ski at a high level into my mid-fifties. I have also referred hundreds of friends, family members, clients, and employees to Egoscue to eliminate pain and regain their ability to engage in the activities they love. The Egoscue Method has proved to be a lifelong method to avoid pain and maintain athleticism!"

—Scott Blanchard,
president, The Ken Blanchard Companies

"I've been suffering from intermittent back problems all my life. Pete Egoscue's method is the first thing I've found that realigns my posture and completely relieves that gnawing pain. I do my Egoscue exercises in just minutes, every single day, and it has changed my life."

—John David Mann, co-author of
the bestselling Go-Giver series

"We have seen firsthand how Pete Egoscue's method has cured people who had suffered with chronic pain for years. He helped transform Sonia from a young mother with debilitating back pain to a strong, confident, active woman. Our entire family and network of friends have relied on The Egoscue Method to help our bodies achieve their original design, thereby freeing us from pain and unleashing our full potential. The same can happen for you. No one knows the body like Pete Egoscue. He is a genius, a marvel, and a movement, and this book can literally and legitimately change our world, one body at a time."

—Sonia and Paul Tudor Jones

"Born from the genius of Pete Egoscue, the simple and effective routines in *Pain Free* are the cutting edge of physical therapy. This book is extraordinary, and I am thrilled to recommend it to anyone who's interested in dramatically increasing the quality of their physical health."

—Tony Robbins, author of
Awaken the Giant Within and *Unlimited Power*

By Pete Egoscue

The Egoscue Method of Health Through Motion

Pain Free

Pain Free at Your PC

Pain Free for Women

Let's Lighten Up

Pain Free Living

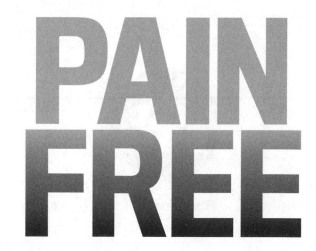

Bantam Books
New York

PETE EGOSCUE

PAIN FREE

A REVOLUTIONARY METHOD FOR STOPPING CHRONIC PAIN

REVISED AND UPDATED
SECOND EDITION

Bantam Books hardcover edition published October 1998, Bantam Books trade paperback edition published July 1999, Bantam Books revised and updated trade paperback second edition published November 2021

Published in the United States by Bantam Books, an imprint of Random House, a division of Penguin Random House LLC, New York.

BANTAM BOOKS and the HOUSE colophon are registered trademarks of Penguin Random House LLC.

Library of Congress Cataloging-in-Publication Data
    Names: Egoscue, Pete, 1945– author.
    Title: Pain free / Pete Egoscue.
    Description: Revised and updated second edition. | New York: Bantam Dell, 2021.
    Identifiers: LCCN 2020048736 (print) | LCCN 2020048737 (ebook) | ISBN 9781101886649 (trade paperback) | ISBN 9780593357767 (ebook)
    Subjects: LCSH: Chronic pain—Exercise therapy.
    Classification: LCC RB127 .E35 2021 (print) | LCC RB127 (ebook) | DDC 616/.0472—dc23
    LC record available at https://lccn.loc.gov/2020048736
    LC ebook record available at https://lccn.loc.gov/2020048737

Printed in the United States of America on acid-free paper

randomhousebooks.com

9th Printing

Book design by George Karabotsos

To all those countless
individuals who have used
The Egoscue Method
for forty-plus years.
You have not only
allowed me to live my dream,
but you have also given me
endless opportunities to
appreciate the magnificence
of the human body.
And, you have given me
daily inspiration about
the power of hope and
the resilience of
the human spirit.

Foreword

"How long has that right shoulder been hurting you?"

These were the first words Pete Egoscue had ever spoken to me. I was a fifteen-year-old sophomore at Torrey Pines High School, north of San Diego, and Pete was at our school to see a Division I football prospect who was a friend of mine. I was the "QB—to be" the following year and was dragged there to throw to my friend so that Pete could evaluate and help my buddy. I had pitched six innings the day before, and although I hadn't told anyone, my shoulder was throbbing in pain.

"How did you know my shoulder was hurting me?" I asked in disbelief.

Pete Egoscue, a former Marine, barked back, "Well, son, it's not duck season in Del Mar . . . is it?"

He was referencing the fact that as my shoulder was killing me, I was struggling to throw any semblance of a spiral. When a ball flutters in football it is referred to as a "duck." His comment was not intended as a compliment. I was young, competitive, and prideful, and I didn't like being embarrassed, so I glared back at the imposing, barrel-chested Marine. He instantly changed his demeanor, smiled at me, and ignoring everyone else on the field asked, "Can I help you?"

Pete took me off to the side and had me do three exercises. Simple exercises. He asked me to stand with my toes angled in and to pull my shoulder blades down and back. He had me lie on a park bench with one leg pulled close to my chest and the other hanging free so that my groin would release. He had me make circles with my arm hanging free, aided by the weight of a nearby rock and gravity. Just as I was thinking, *What the heck is this guy doing,* he finished things off by asking me to do a downward dog. This was 1987—doing yoga poses was the epitome of a high school football player's most embarrassing nightmare.

Pete's entire sequence had taken maybe three minutes, but everyone was eagerly wanting to get back to the workout. I got up and Pete's bark returned: "Now go throw a damn spiral."

My shoulder had been so painful during the preceding throws that I was really not looking forward to attempting another, but I had to for my buddy. I took my drop, unleashed the ball, and braced myself for the pain that had followed my previous throws. But the pain never came. I watched as my spiral sailed downfield—it was the best ball I had ever thrown.

I looked at Pete and smirked. He had embarrassed me, so I had no intention of giving him any credit. He smiled and said, "Again."

I dropped back and unleashed another ball. I again watched, completely free of pain, as my spiral sailed smoothly downfield. If my previous throw hadn't been my best ever, this throw surely would have been. I looked at him and asked, "What did you do to me?"

He said, "I didn't do anything, you did."

Pete explained to me that nothing was wrong with my shoulder. Rather, the position of my shoulder had gotten out of whack, and he simply had to teach me to reposition it. I didn't exactly understand, but I knew with certainty that I felt no pain and was throwing better than I ever had. In three minutes, he unlocked my body, unleashing my potential to optimize whatever talents the good Lord and my parents had blessed me with.

I went home and told my mom and dad about my experience.

My dad had already heard of Pete and looked into things before sitting me down for a chat the next week. He told me that Pete typically didn't work with people my age and would do so only if I committed to three things: (1) always be on time, (2) do the "menus" and workouts exactly as Pete prescribed, and (3) never be late. I was a teenager and lightheartedly thought, *Well, that is really only two rules,* but my dad was far more serious. He felt it was a little much to have someone making house calls to see a fifteen-year-old, but he also knew that my dream was to be a professional athlete. And he knew that I was willing to work to achieve that dream. My dad said we would give it a trial run but Pete's three rules were his three rules.

It's almost thirty-five years later now, and a lot has changed. I earned a scholarship to Stanford University. I was drafted, I was signed, and I played both professional baseball and professional football. My ultimate career path followed my passion and took me to the NFL, where I had a fifteen-year career. I captained the Tampa Bay Buccaneers in Super Bowl XXXVII, made nine Pro Bowls, and was a four-time All Pro. Fewer than ten players in league history have been named to the Ring of Honor in two different franchises. I am one of those players for both the Tampa Bay Buccaneers and the Denver Broncos. I was inducted into the Pro Football Hall of Fame. I have lived a charmed life. I despise talking about myself. That is how I was raised, and more so, that is my personality. But I list these accomplishments in gratitude because in addition to my coaches, my teammates, my parents, and my wife, Pete Egoscue was very much responsible for my success and helping me achieve my dreams.

Pete Egoscue taught me how to work. Moreover, he taught me how to "outwork" my competition. He taught me mental toughness and showed me that my body was strong and resilient. He taught me, and so many other athletes at all levels, that "your body won't let you down, your mind will." He helped me unleash every ounce of athletic ability that I had. By pushing me in the off-seasons since I was fifteen years old, he taught me the mental advantage that you have by knowing you can outlast your competition. The fourth quarter was always my friend. As my competition was getting worn out, I was just getting going.

Pete taught me that my body was more than capable of taking on the rigors of the NFL. I played a very physical brand of football in an era when that was how you played the game. People have always asked, then and now, "How did your body last playing that way for fifteen years?" I know that there is no way my body would have allowed me to perform and last that long if not for my work with Pete.

Quite simply, Pete is the most brilliant person that I have ever encountered when it comes to the human body and unleashing its vast potential. That is why today, in my role as the general manager of the San Francisco 49ers, Pete and The Egoscue Method are an integral element of our Health and Performance team.

So I encourage you to enjoy this book. It is such a cliché to say that this will change your life, but this will change your life. You will feel better, stand taller, and be able to enjoy more activities. You will be able to sustain a quality of life that so many believe is not feasible or available to them. It is available to you, and this book will give you the tools to do that and live a healthy, happy pain-free life.

John Lynch
October 2021
Santa Clara, California

Contents

Foreword... xi

A Disclaimer About Disclaimers............... xvii

Introduction... xix

Chapter 1:
The Modern Pain Epidemic......................... 3

Chapter 2:
Movement: Our Survival Superpower 12

Chapter 3:
Our Magnificent Design............................ 24

Chapter 4:
Understanding Pain: Our Perception
Versus Reality... 35

Chapter 5:
The Egoscue Method: A Life in Balance...... 45

Chapter 6:
Feet and Ankles:
Our Musculoskeletal Sole......................... 56

Chapter 7:
Knees: The Biology of Benders 90

Chapter 8:
The Hip and the Pelvis:
Central Command.................................... 120

Chapter 9:
The Spine: Our Backbone of Function....... 152

Chapter 10:
The Shoulders: The Mobility King............ 182

Chapter 11:
Head and Neck: The Crown of Balance...... 210

Chapter 12:
Elbows, Wrists, and Hands:
Elegant Efficiency.................................. 240

Conclusion: My Parting Wish for You....... 270

Acknowledgments.................................. 273

Notes.. 275

Index.. 277

A Disclaimer About Disclaimers

It has become obligatory for health books to carry a legal disclaimer. You've read them: "The following advice is not intended to substitute for the advice of a physician . . ." And they go on to recommend that you consult a doctor before embarking on whatever program is being offered. They conclude with the author and publisher disclaiming any legal responsibility for adverse consequences.

If you need the disclaimer's protection, close this book and leave the pages unread.

My working principle as an author and exercise therapist is that the most important consultation is the one you have with yourself. Healthcare starts with personal responsibility.

Introduction

A number of decades ago, I wrote my first book talking about the wonder of the human body. Since that time, the world has undergone an amazing change—a dramatic acceleration of technology.

The marvels of human creativity have enhanced our abilities in every aspect of daily life, except one—our bodies. As the requirements of existence depend less and less on our ability to move (we live at our desks, in our cars, and on our couches), our health and physical capabilities have declined. Chronic pain has become the number one issue in our healthcare system, and it has perplexed and frustrated the medical community for decades.

This frustration has led to a variety of treatment options and interventions, drug therapies, physical therapy of all types, surgeries, braces, and a large number of research studies trying to determine the best way to alleviate pain.

All of these approaches begin with a seemingly logical premise—the site of the pain is the place to treat. In other words, the source of the pain and the cause of the pain are one and the same.

The problem? That's simply not true when it comes to cases of sustained chronic pain. Why is that? Let's use the example of a broken arm. An accident happens, you break a bone, and you feel pain and discomfort. As the bone heals, the pain gradually subsides. Cause and effect: Bone damage causes pain. Bone healing alleviates pain.

Next, let's take a look at a herniated disc—a problem that's a common source of the most prevalent pain in our country, back pain. The disc—as it slips or bulges out of its place in the spine—doesn't heal. The pain comes and goes. But the broken bone healed, so why doesn't the herniated disc?

The answer: Healing chronic pain is about understanding its cause. An event caused the broken bone. That event is over. The body, as a living organism, begins the process of healing the damage caused by the event. The event was the action—or stimulus—that resulted in the break. Since that stimulus is no longer acting on the bone, the bone can heal. The disc does not heal because the stimulus that produced the herniation is still present. The body's natural process to repair tissue doesn't work because the cause—the stimulus—is still present and active.

This is the core principle of *Pain Free:* You can heal pain only when you identify and treat its cause. And that cause may not be so obvious. As a living organism, the body is in a constant state of cell renewal. Not being in that state is a sign of disease or system imbalance.

This book is about helping you find and treat the cause, so you can allow your body to heal and thrive.

That cause: muscle imbalance.

This book represents more than forty years of confirmation that muscle imbalance is the cause of the maladies producing chronic pain. Restoring our naturally designed balance solves the problem and cures the pain.

This reality, as true and powerful as it is, presents a modern challenge to you. We as a culture have become convinced that humans are fragile, easily broken, and limited in our abilities to achieve and maintain perfect health. We are told repeatedly by well-meaning experts that our bodies are so complex that only they can determine health or treatment options and outcomes.

You are challenged not to rely on your own wisdom, instincts, experience, and beliefs. Your self-reliance is important only if it is supported by expert guidance.

This book is about you and your expertise. My experience as a postural therapist has taught me that you know more about your body than any expert, including me.

The challenge for me, the author, is to provide evidence and common sense in order for you not only to believe in your own wisdom, but more important, also to act on that wisdom. I hope the book achieves this goal.

If you will trust yourself and grasp the simple, brilliant, functional capabilities of your body, your transformation will confirm that a balanced musculoskeletal system produces the energy and capacity for you to lead a well-lived life—pain free.

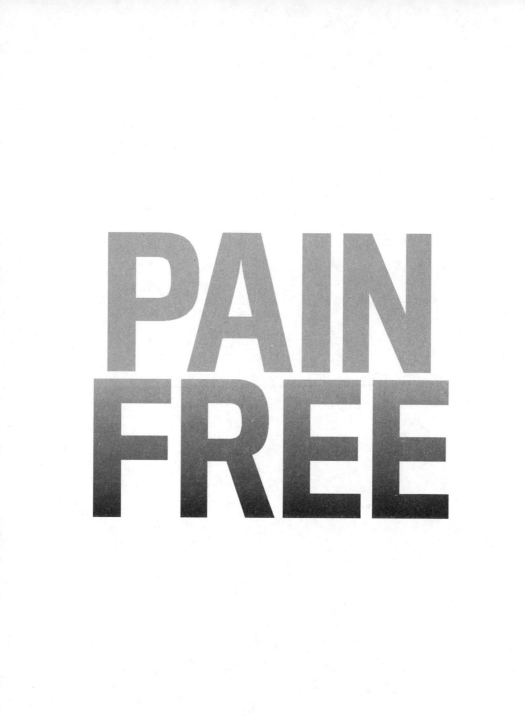

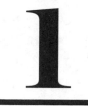

The Modern Pain Epidemic

Pain causes more of a burden on our society today than it has at any other point during history. Musculoskeletal pain—the type that comes from the bones, joints, muscles, and nerves—affects more than 50 percent of the adult population in the United States. Musculoskeletal problems are the leading cause of global disability. And despite all the advances of modern medicine, that burden has been steadily growing for the last several decades.

Pain is often portrayed as one of the human body's most enigmatic curses—one with no shortage of purported cures. We have wave-your-wand magic potions, glitzy technology, and fancy diagnoses. We have developed pain-killing medications that are so strong and addictive, they have become the cause of one of the worst drug problems in humanity's history.

And yet, the problem persists. Pain continues to limit—even ruin—millions of lives. Why? What I know is this: we have just about everything backward when it comes to how we understand, prevent, and treat pain.

Our pain problem persists because our modern environment and the approaches of modern medicine have not addressed the only thing that can stop pain—the *source* of it.

Here is the funny thing—and what I have learned over my four decades of working with people in varying degrees of pain like you. The answer to this complex problem is simple.

You.

You have the power to fix your pain—if you stop fearing it and learn to understand it. In doing so, you will learn to trust yourself and take back control of your journey.

Before we get into the intricacies of the body in the next sections, let's think about the big picture—and how we got into this painful mess to begin with.

Modern Society's Triad of Pain

When I look at today's society and compare it to the society of a half century ago, I see three key differences that are fueling our pain epidemic.

We Live in Fear. Today's modern culture has given us a lot of great things (I like playing on my phone as much as the next person), yet there are unintended consequences to living in a hyperfast world. Many of us have robbed ourselves of the fundamental belief that our bodies have the ability to bounce back.

Growing up, you probably remember banging your knee and having a parent or coach say, "Shake it off, work it out, you're going to be fine." That wasn't just tough love. That was an unconscious acknowledgment of our innate resilience and the body's incredible capacity to heal all on its own. As kids, we viewed the pain from our banged knee as a message that our body was still healing.

But something happens as we grow up—something that changes our innate understanding of pain's purpose. We begin to fear pain, viewing it as a problem to address rather than a message to understand. A problem requires a solution—a pill, a procedure, an expert—to make it all disappear.

In the end, this has *hurt* us.

We no longer collectively have the self-reliance and emotional capacity to empower our own bodies to help us. We have become environmentally cautious and risk averse, and therefore, when something hurts, we do not intuitively know how to handle it. We have lost our childhood intuition to see pain as a message. Instead, we are quick to jump to worst-case-scenario problems and to look for solutions outside ourselves—from pills, procedures, and experts. We must relearn that intuitive self-reliance if we are to be successful in our battle against pain.

Treating Symptoms Is Not the Same as Fixing Causes. Pain is the result of a complex mix of anatomy, biology, and neurology with no universal fix. Despite a healthcare system that offers countless treatment options, relief is frequently marginal and sporadic. Consistent, complete relief is all too often elusive. Surgery isn't a guaranteed fix for many problems and carries the risk of damaging the fragile ecosystem of the human body. Painkillers may be up to the task of hiding the pain, but they are the medical equivalent of a masquerade party. They cover up the symptom, but they don't address the root cause of whatever triggered the curse-inducing agony to begin with.

Modern musculoskeletal medicine uses technology to find and fix problems on a micro level. Let's use back pain as an example. This is one of our most pervasive pains with no accepted one-size-fits-all approach. Perhaps your MRI shows a herniated disc that is compressing a nearby nerve root. Plenty of interventions have the potential to relieve that pain. But there are important questions that are often left unasked.

What caused the herniated disc?

What is happening to cause such an abnormal stress that the disc was forced to herniate?

These questions need to be explored and answered to find and fix the root cause of your problem. This requires a macro look at the body rather than a micro focus on the location of the pain.

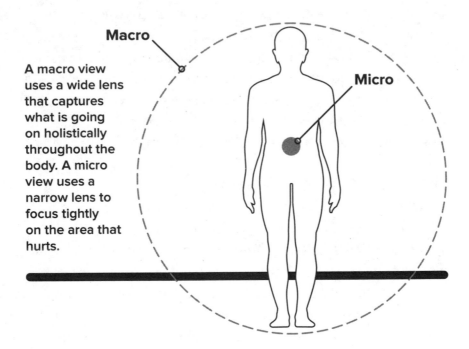

Macro

A macro view uses a wide lens that captures what is going on holistically throughout the body. A micro view uses a narrow lens to focus tightly on the area that hurts.

Micro

We use MRIs, CT scans, and X-rays with more frequency than ever before. We have more information readily available at our fingertips than any previous era. Yet pain is more pervasive than at any other point in history. Why? Because the information (or in medical terms, the diagnosis) provided by these technologies addresses only the micro issue. An MRI provides information about only a small portion of your musculoskeletal system.

Paths to Pain Free

Dr. Paul Hodgson, New Wave Chiropractic Center

Dr. Paul Hodgson has always been an athlete. He played ball sports when he was younger—basketball, football, rugby. Now he's more into yoga, rock climbing, and endurance sports. Over the years, he's suffered from acute injuries that turned chronic—that is, problem spots that never really healed, so they would always get reaggravated and reinjured.

In addition, he's had poor posture his whole life. "Being a chiropractor with bad posture is like being a dentist with bad teeth—in my mind, unacceptable," he says.

When Brian Bradley, a VP at Egoscue, took his son to Hodgson for treatment of an injury, they got talking about posture, and Hodgson took a look at Bradley's spine.

"When I saw his spine on an X-ray, I had noticed that he had one of the best spines I had ever seen for his age, in terms of degeneration, disc spacing, joint spacing, and bone health," he says. "That piqued my interest."

Hodgson began doing E-cises, the exercises of The Egoscue Method, and noticed a whole lot of changes in his body—including being more aware of his posture and body movement (he's already very aware as a chiropractor and yoga practitioner). He now does all kinds of movements without worrying about getting injured, and he tells his clients about adding E-cises to help their pains.

"My body is visibly and functionally very different and probably the strongest it's ever been. I'm thirty-six and definitely getting older," he says, "but my body feels like it's getting stronger."

The narrowness of that focus is compounded by the fact that the images are static—completely absent is the impact of movement on the visualized structures. If the root cause of the pain falls outside that micro lens, it likely will never be discovered.

For example, elbow pain can originate from poor shoulder position. Back pain can come from weak hips. These causes are not going to show up on a micro-focused MRI aimed at your elbow or back. We must zoom out and consider the macro view to understand and address the source of our pain.

It's Not Just Biological. It's Environmental. More and more, our worlds have zero physical motion. At work, at home, and in our recreational environments, routine movement is becoming a thing of the past. Just think about desks and cars, smartphones and videogames, televisions and computers. Think about how many hours we spend each day hunched over, crunched up, and jumbled into an anatomical tangle of tendons and tissues.

Food and water are available literally at our fingertips. With the click of a button we can have groceries delivered. Go one step further to takeout delivery, and all the movement necessary for cooking is eliminated. Heck, one of the fastest-growing recreational activities is *watching* people play videogames. We are paying money to sit in packed arenas and watch other people sit. These motionless scenarios play out over and over, everywhere, every day.

Our bodies were meant to get up and move, but collectively we no longer do it. Your commitment to movement will provide you the foundation for living pain free.

The Pain Cycle

These three pain problems—especially when intertwined— are the reasons why pain so frequently becomes an inescapable cycle of suffering.

Fear causes us to have tunnel vision about our pain—we become micro-focused on what hurts. Modern musculoskeletal medicine reinforces that focus with micro tests and diagnoses that fail to capture our macro environment. Without an understanding of our macro environment, the cause of our pain remains an unsolved mystery. That uncertainty feeds right into our fear. This self-perpetuating cycle can become difficult to escape.

Even if you have a proper diagnosis for your pain—a herniated disc, a migraine, arthritis—the therapy you apply can't address a root cause you don't understand. Without that understanding and a fix for pain's underlying origin, the uncertainty of when and why the pain will return becomes crippling. You become scared still, quite literally afraid to move. That is the cycle we need to break ASAP.

The Vicious Cycle of Modern Pain

We live in a motionless world.

We develop pain we don't understand.

Without self-reliance, we skip self-help and immediately seek help from outside experts.

We get a quick fix to our immediate problem that often fails to address the root cause of our pain.

The pain continues and because we don't understand it, we become fearful and scared still.

HOW TODAY'S PAIN IS DIFFERENT

Forty Years Ago

In the 1920s, manual workers outnumbered knowledge workers by a ratio of 2:1. By 1980, that ratio was reversed. Although humans were spending more time sitting and less time moving at work, technology was less pervasive than it is now, which meant movement was still relatively commonplace even in office jobs (walking across the hallway to make a copy, taking the stairs to a meeting, strolling a few blocks to pick up lunch).

Activities of daily living and recreational activities still largely centered on movement, so even the most sedentary workers were commonly moving outside the workplace.

When people felt pain, it was a result of being tight and stiff. Muscles like movement—they start to feel stiff and tight when they go for long periods of time without motion. The increasing prevalence of sitting reduced the frequency that muscles were put to work.

Today

In today's society, movement as a requirement for survival is largely a thing of the past. Technology has changed the way we work, play, and carry out our everyday, necessary life activities. For virtually every imaginable activity, there is a technological solution that eliminates or reduces the amount of movement required to accomplish our objective.

Today, we move so little that we have moved beyond the "stiffness" of yesteryear. Our muscles are called into action so infrequently that most musculoskeletal pain is the result of muscle weakness. When our muscles don't have the necessary strength to carry out a desired movement, we start to compensate, creating instability and imbalance that results in pain.

Our challenge today results from the complexity of our compensations for these underlying muscle weaknesses. The pain that results rarely occurs at the location of weakness. Instead we feel pain somewhere else—the result of some abnormal strain or stress that results from the compensation for our underlying weakness.

People could treat their pain by stretching or moving their muscles to decrease their stiffness. They had confidence in themselves. They understood that being stiff and tight was a consequence of infrequent movement. But because *some* type of movement was still commonplace, most people were not weak. Movement was not feared. Rather, people trusted that moving their muscles would help their discomfort and pain.

Because today's chain of events is more complex and less predictable than the pain of forty years ago, we have lost confidence in our ability to understand and fix our pain. We focus on the area that hurts (duh—that's what catches our attention), but we completely miss the underlying muscle weakness that caused the problem to begin with.

Modern musculoskeletal medicine reinforces this focus with imaging and high-tech diagnostics that focus on the area of pain. Temporary fixes for pain help the area of focus, but the source remains unaddressed—leaving us vulnerable to more pain and frustration. Our lack of understanding creates a vicious cycle of mistrust in ourselves and the "experts" we look to for help.

RESULT: People had the self-reliance to treat and resolve their pain because they understood what caused it and what they needed to do to address that underlying cause.

RESULT: Our pain persists because of a lack of understanding about why pain occurs. This triggers a cycle of mistrust, uncertainty, and frustration that diminishes our self-reliance.

2

Movement: Our Survival Superpower

We are designed to move. Life may seem challenging to define in a universally accepted way, but all the characteristics frequently used in definitions involve movement. Growth, reproduction, environmental responsiveness, ability to change and adapt—none of these things is static in nature.

Movement is necessary for life.

So much so, that we have an entire sensory system dedicated exclusively to helping us move well. We are preprogrammed to sense stimuli within our environment and respond with action that increases the likelihood of our survival. This kinesthetic sense is dependent on our ability to perceive the position and movement of our body in space. This incoming sensory information allows us to adapt and maximize our function within our current environment.

Refining our kinesthetic sense requires practice. An expert wilderness guide learns to recognize storm clouds on the horizon by spending day after day wandering around in the mountains. A financial expert learns to recognize advantageous trends in the stock market through years of trading experience. Mastering our ability to sense and respond to our environment requires repetitive opportunities to practice that skill.

Movement is how we practice. During movement, our body receives feedback from the environment from which we learn to optimize our function. A young child learning to walk readily illustrates how we refine our kinesthetic sense. Initially, the child will fail and fall over and over, more closely resembling a tranquilized elephant or drunken sailor than a coordinated human being. It is a survival marvel that despite being born without the inherent knowledge that, when falling forward, putting one's hands out to break the fall is protective, we have survived as a species for this long. It does not take many faceplants for a young child to learn that lesson.

With each early attempt and subsequent fall, the child is learning which actions are helpful and which actions are harmful to its efforts to stay upright. But that learning process is not linear. After learning to stand, an exorbitant amount of bum-flopping follows. Ultimately the child will learn the balance necessary to stay upright and master the art of bending its pudgy knees to sit down more gracefully. Until then, thank God for padded diapers. The child will plop backward time and time again. Concerned parents will question how many times the little one is going to make the same mistake. But those same parents will soon find themselves wishing their little one would master subsequent challenges just a touch slower.

Each challenge increases the child's sensitivity to feedback, allowing the child to learn faster and move on to new mistakes, correcting subsequent missteps far more quickly. Each failure gives the child yet another nugget of knowledge that moves them closer to success. Ongoing environmental interactions make us hypersensitive to feedback, allowing us to more readily recognize and learn from our mistakes.

Early failures do not leave young children feeling fearful, fragile, or inadequate. In fact, anyone who has spent time around young children will say the exact opposite. Despite bumbling about in their environment, young children are empowered by, and all too frequently, overconfident in their newly acquired movement skills. Bum flops and faceplants hurt, but children do not fear pain. To children, pain provides a message about what went wrong. They course-correct and move on. Each challenge and subsequent success instills resilience, a trait we all too often lose touch with as adults. Stationary lifestyles result in fewer interactions with our environment, and our sensitivity to feedback dwindles. We slowly stop recognizing and learning from our shortcomings, and our confidence in our innate ability to course-correct disappears.

Adaptation—the Body's Limitless Learning Potential

A child's journey to walking is the first of many learning curves in this life that revolve around gravity. Gravity is the most pervasive stimulus in our environment. Efficiently responding to gravity is a prerequisite for our survival on Earth, and our body has numerous tailor-made adaptations to this inescapable stimulus.

We have adapted and evolved to the degree that ongoing interactions with gravity are necessary for our health. Consider what happens to astronauts during long space voyages. Astro-

Paths to Pain Free

Dr. Heather Sandison, Founder and Medical Director, North County Natural Medicine and the Marama Experience

As a massage therapist in her early twenties, Dr. Heather Sandison encountered lots of clients suffering with chronic pain. A handful told them about their success with The Egoscue Method, so she started to work with us.

What was most helpful, she says, was "empowering clients to own the process and feel in charge of their own body. Clients are the ones making the changes and getting out of pain."

Sandison says that what's important is knowing the relationship between the physical and psychological. "A big part of what we were doing as postural therapists was not only showing people how to help align their bodies and live pain free but showing them they were capable of doing it for themselves," she says. "They didn't need someone to fix them. They just needed to show up and do the menu and their pain could resolve."

---

nauts can lose up to 20 percent of their muscle mass after just one week in space. Bones also weaken. Without the stimulus of bearing weight, the minerals necessary for strong bones are reabsorbed by the body. This is most pronounced in the hips, pelvis, and spine—the areas where most of our weight is distributed down here on Earth.

The impact of a zero gravity environment is not limited to the musculoskeletal system. Gravity makes fluid accumulate in the lower part of the body, and humans have evolved in response to that stimulus. We have systems that return blood and fluid to the heart and brain even while we stand. These systems continue to work in outer space. Without the counterbalancing effect of gravity, astronauts frequently accumulate fluid in the upper body, which causes blurry vision and balance problems.

The heart muscle also weakens as the need to maintain blood pressure is decreased without the effects of gravity.

The good news for astronauts is that these changes reverse themselves upon return to Earth. Reapply the stimulus of gravity and the body will adapt to survive on Earth once again. Our body is brilliantly designed to sense our environment and respond to that environment with actions that facilitate the movements necessary for survival.

The Human Musculoskeletal System —Perfectly Adapted to Earth

On Earth, for gravity to exert a positive influence on the body, the skeleton must be vertically aligned. Humans are designed as symmetrical bipeds, which means we are designed to move about on two extremities and the left side of our body should identically mirror the right side. We should be symmetrical from side to side. There are four major load joints on each side of the body—the shoulder, hip, knee, and ankle. The spine runs along the midline of the body. These joints, and the muscles that surround them, are designed to hold the weight—or load—of the body vertically.

Gravity is providing a continuous stimulus to which the body must respond in order to stay upright. Vertical alignment of the load joints minimizes the work required to stabilize the body against the downward pull of gravity. The body is most efficient when the spine, ankles, knees, hips, and shoulders rest along parallel lines.

Joints are areas where two bones meet. Bones do what muscles tell them to do. Therefore, the position of our bones and joints is controlled by our muscles. Vertical alignment of our joints is facilitated through a coordinated effort of our muscles known as dynamic tension.

Perfect Symmetry

There are four major load joints on each side of the body—the shoulder, the hip, the knee, and the ankle. These joints, and the muscles that surround them, are designed to hold the weight—or load— of the body vertically. These joints should ideally be positioned along a vertical line along either side of the body. When these joints (and the spine) rest along parallel lines, the body is most efficient.

Shoulder

Hip

Knee

Ankle

Throughout our musculoskeletal system, most of our muscles exist in pairs with opposite functions. The quadriceps extends the knee; the hamstring flexes the knee. The back muscles straighten the spine; the abdominal muscles bend the spine.

Opposing muscle pairs provide the critical balance that holds our joints in the positions necessary for ideal musculo-skeletal function. This dynamic tension holds our joints in an aligned, vertical column. If the dynamic tension between opposing muscles is lost, the joints will shift from this aligned position. This makes the body less efficient and decreases our overall stability and mobility.

Our balanced state of dynamic tension and vertical loading is critically important when it comes to musculoskele-tal wear and tear. Our musculoskeletal system absorbs huge amounts of force from the weight of our body as we move and stand. When the body is properly aligned, the stress on our joints, bones, and muscles is minimized. When the body falls out of alignment, our joints, bones, and muscles become subject to abnormal stress and strain, increasing the likelihood of injury and pain.

The essential nature of balance to our function is perhaps illustrated nowhere more clearly than with the human spine. Just like our ability to walk on two legs, the human spine is unique in the animal world. We are the only species that has a characteristic S-shape to our spine, and its formation is unques-tionably an adaptive consequence of the demand to hold our body upright.

Our S-curve perfectly balances the need for rigidity to hold the human stable in the upright position with the need for flexibility to facilitate movement. Our pelvis is more mobile than that of other animal species. This mobility increases stride length and makes two-legged ambulation more energy efficient. The S-curve of our spine plays a critical role in this mobility. Our spinal curve prevents us from falling over by keeping the weight of our upper body balanced over our mobile pelvis. Loss of that critical S-curve not only hinders our mobility but also disrupts our stability and balance in the upright position.

The Magic of Movement

Balance is critical to our musculoskeletal system's ability to function efficiently and with minimal wear and tear. Movement is required to maintain our balanced state. The "use it or lose it" mantra rings very true for living organisms. Humans are no exception; every one of our interconnected body systems requires movement to function properly.

Muscles require use to maintain flexibility and contractility. Bones require loading to maintain strength. The heart requires resistance to maintain its endurance and efficiency. The lungs require expansion to maintain compliance. The intestines require peristalsis to facilitate digestion and absorb nutrients. The brain requires cardiac contraction and respiration to facilitate the movement of cerebrospinal fluid needed for proper neurological function.

Interestingly, today's humans are among the minority of living creatures that are not moved, at least on some occasions, by natural external forces. For us, there is no drifting with the tide or gliding on currents of air. Today's society does not regularly require that we hunt for survival or wander in search of shelter to escape inclement weather. We either make the choice to move ourselves or we perish. It is that simple.

Without movement, our systems function at a suboptimal level. Our capacity for existence slowly declines. As a living organism, we are in a constant state of growth and rebirth. This renewal requires energy—energy that is derived from the movement-centered function of our body systems. In scientific terms, this energy is referred to as metabolic rate. Generally speaking, the higher the metabolic rate, the healthier the human being. Without adequate movement, our body functions at less-than-ideal levels and our metabolic rate falls. We simply have less energy to invest in growth and renewal, meaning we age and ultimately die faster.

Unintended Consequences of Our Modern Motionless Existence

As our society has grown more sedentary, we have lost the connection between joy and movement. Muscles in motion act as the conductor of a biological orchestra that instantly elevates mental and physical health. We know that exercise improves our endurance, strength, and cardiovascular health, but movement is also directly connected to feelings of hope, happiness, connection, and confidence.

Exercise is the most demanding activity the brain encounters. Yes—you read that correctly. From a metabolic perspective, exercising places more demands on the brain than reading, writing, or playing chess. Movement unlocks a built-in superpharmacy that triggers the release of hormones, neurotransmitters (molecules that behave as our body's chemical version of bike messengers), and proteins that affect energy levels, mood, brain function, social engagement, and outlook.

Movement triggers the release of endorphins and cannabinoids. These messengers tell our body to decrease stress levels, increase pain tolerance, boost pleasure, and increase feelings of well-being. Endorphins also increase our sense of connection, increasing the pleasure we derive from social interactions and strengthening the bonds we form with others. Humans are inherently social creatures, and endorphins help us form meaningful connections that fight feelings of loneliness and isolation.

Movement also increases the production of dopamine and the release of myokines. Dopamine is a neurotransmitter that increases feelings of motivation, fortitude, and courage. Myokines are proteins associated with improved memory and learning.

It is no coincidence that as our society has become more and more sedentary, levels of depression, anxiety, suicide, and drug addiction have skyrocketed. In becoming motionless, we

Paths to Pain Free

John Cook, Head Coach, University of Nebraska Women's Volleyball

When John Cook became assistant coach of the US men's national volleyball team in the early 1990s, he was charged with coming up with a plan to keep the men strong and healthy. This was crucial because the team had a lot of older guys (in their thirties) and they had a brutal travel schedule (often bouncing weekend to weekend from the US to Europe, back to the US, then to Asia).

Cook had heard about Egoscue, and he witnessed and joined in workouts with many elite athletes, like John Lynch of the San Francisco 49ers. One time, he remembers doing a brutal run up a steep hill where partners had to piggyback-carry each other up the hill. His partner—who had a history of back pain that couldn't be fixed even though he had traveled all over the country seeking a solution—carried him up with no problem. He had been training for a month in The Egoscue Method, and that crushing piggyback carry didn't hurt his back at all. "That really resonated with me," he says.

To this day, Cook still uses The Egoscue Method to help himself stay in shape and as part of his workouts with the Huskers volleyball team.

One time, one of his All-American players ruptured a disc. All of the surgeons wanted to operate and shut her down. But after three days of Egoscue treatments, she was healed and went on to continue her career as one of the greatest Nebraska athletes ever.

Another time, one of his US men's players started warming up for a match abroad and went down as if someone had shot him—his legs wouldn't work and his back was frozen. The trainer got on the phone and talked the player through several Egoscue exercises. "By the end of the day, he was great and back in practice the next day," says Cook, who does exercises with the team (which he says is the reason he can be a physical coach, moving throughout practices with his team).

"It's all about posture, and Pete has figured out how to get people back in good posture and have things work the way they're supposed to work," Cook says.

throw away the key necessary to unlock our built-in vault of energy, purpose, and well-being.

The loss of movement and joy is compounded by the ever-increasing prevalence of technology in our world. Don't get me wrong—technology has been hugely beneficial in the advancement of civilization, but it has not come without a price. Phones are a major contributor to our motionless environment. The average person checks their phone almost sixty times per day, spending more than three hours staring down at a four-inch screen. Text messages and emails have replaced telephone calls and in-person communication, increasing our sense of social isolation. Smartphones also make it ridiculously easy to carelessly consume our free time. Three hours is 20 percent of our waking day—no wonder we feel like we "have no time." Imagine how much we could improve our lives if we spent just a fraction of that time moving our bodies rather than our thumbs.

Our sedentary nature has also made us increasingly risk averse. Less movement means more infrequent interactions with our environment. Our kinesthetic sense becomes rusty, decreasing our environmental awareness and leaving us feeling less confident in our ability to survive in our surroundings. We have slowly lost the self-confidence necessary to trust ourselves to persevere and succeed in the face of uncertainty. Instead, we attempt to eliminate perceived risk and uncertainty by creating a false sense of security and control.

The problem is that our world is a very unpredictable place. There is much that we simply cannot control. Being human is a risky business. Everything we do involves risk. There is risk in the air we breathe, the water we drink, and the food we eat. There is risk in driving a car, falling in love, and having a child.

Today, we recoil from spontaneous changes in our environment rather than responding to them. We are consistently choosing *flight* over *fight* because we no longer have the courage to confront uncertainty head on. In always choosing flight,

Dr. Dustin Dillberg, Acupuncturist, Pain Free Kauai

Dr. Dustin Dillberg has always been on a path to study Eastern medicine. After he was in a car accident when he was young, his father used acupuncture to help with related migraines. As early as junior high, he knew he wanted to study East Asian medicine. As part of his medical schooling, he studied Egoscue—and was a bit skeptical ("It sounded too good to be true," he says). But he immersed himself in it and saw how it could help people as part of a multifunctional approach to healing.

"Every bit of our being depends on movement and moving from the correct start positions. It helps people get to the sources of their imbalance—movement and posture always play a role," he says.

we lose touch with our resilience, a trait that can be developed only by persevering through challenging situations.

We got to this point by actively engaging with our environment. Throughout history, our body used movement to learn about our surroundings and empower us with adaptations that facilitated survival. With diminishing confidence in our ability to respond and survive, the possibility of a bad outcome becomes paralyzing. This is compounded by the fact that modern society makes us hyperaware of bad outcomes, even if those bad outcomes are exceedingly rare. Fear drives us to further recoil from our environment in the name of safety and certainty. The self-empowerment found in coping, pushing back, and enduring all but disappears.

If there is one thing I have learned with certainty over the last forty years, it is this. I may be able to help you eliminate your pain by correcting your imbalance and weakness, but the real power comes from enabling you to return to a life of movement. That is where the real magic begins—and it has nothing to do with me.

3

Our Magnificent Design

My hope is that by the time you reach this stage of the book, that little voice in your head is saying something along the lines of "Damn, my body does a lot of crazy complicated and cool things that I never even think about." If you are hearing that little voice—hallelujah! If you aren't, well, you will just have to settle for my voice screaming the sentiment for now. I am making this point for a reason: recognizing the body's built-in brilliance and power is a key stop on the ride to being pain free.

For me, that reality hit me like a freight train in 1969.

The doctors thought I was unconscious—a reasonable assumption in an intensive care ward of a US hospital ship filled with newly arrived Vietnam combat casualties. They stopped at the cot next to mine, where an army captain moaned in agony. He had been shot in the stomach several days before. The soldier was so badly hurt, he never slept, never talked to anyone, never fell into the merciful arms of silence. There was only the stark, unremitting sound of a man in pain, punctuated by the beeping of heart monitors.

The doctors looked at his chart and made a brief examination of his wound. One of them asked, "Think he'll make it?" I heard the clipboard that held the man's medical record drop back into its holder. I wanted to turn my head to see if they were talking about me, but I couldn't manage it. Too many tubes and too much pain of my own.

The other doctor answered with such a matter-of-fact tone that today I imagine him shrugging as he said, "You either get well or you die."

The young captain died a couple of days later. For forty-plus years, I've been thinking about the captain and what the doctor said. The comment struck me then, as it does now, with the force of a profound truth. The doctor, whether he was aware of it or not, was recognizing that there comes a point when modern medical techniques must give way to the body's own inner logic, mechanisms, and intentions. Despite all the hardware, surgical talent, antibiotics, and painkillers, either you get well or you die.

This is not fatalism, blind faith, or passivity. It is a confirmation and celebration of the body's capacity to maintain health and life, independent of outside intervention that would substitute technology and technical know-how for this ineffable power. The human body not only controls the ultimate transition from life to death but, in the meantime, manages the process we call health and healing. Today, technology and techniques have become so intrusive that they run the risk of overpowering the body's own role in health and healing. And that is a tragedy. Ultimately, there can be neither health nor healing if the body is denied its commanding role in making us well.

With regard to musculoskeletal pain, that commanding role starts with the ingenuity and strength of our musculoskeletal system. The designed interactions of our muscles, bones, and joints are intricately complex, yet simultaneously perfectly suited to our needs.

Simply put, our musculoskeletal system is designed to function in a state of balance. A balanced musculoskeletal system is symmetrical from side to side. An unbalanced musculoskeletal system results from muscle dysfunction. Such dysfunction occurs because of imbalance in muscle strength and flexibility. In an unbalanced musculoskeletal system, the right side of the body will not precisely mirror the left side. This unbalanced, dysfunctional state limits our ability to move, increases the wear and tear on our bones, muscles, and joints, and costs us valuable energy.

Shy of some type of acute trauma, musculoskeletal pain is the result of muscle dysfunction—a change that creates imbalance and disrupts our side-to-side symmetry. To eliminate pain, we must eliminate dysfunction. Without dysfunction, we will return to our balanced, symmetric design, capable of pain-free, limitless motion. But in order to understand how to restore our balance and function, we first need to understand how it was lost.

Pain as an Adaptive Consequence

The human body has an incredible ability to adapt. The body is continuously responding to stimuli and making changes to match its environment. From the instant the human fetus first kicks or shifts its position in the womb, it is moving in reaction to its environment—and it will continue to do so for the rest of its life as long as the environment provides one key ingredient—stimulus.

Stimulus can be external or internal. External stimuli arise from the environment that surrounds our body. Examples include a predator chasing you through the woods, a cold rain that causes you to seek shelter, or an uneven sidewalk that forces you to quickly adjust your step. Internal stimuli arise from

A Balanced System

Functional and Balanced

Dysfunctional and Imbalanced

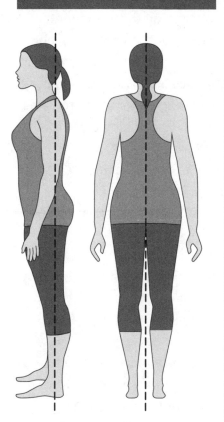

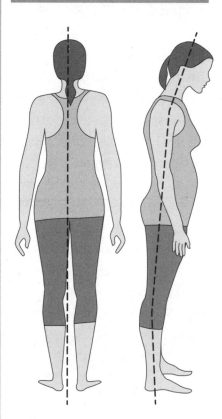

When we are balanced, our right and left sides appear as mirror images across the center line of our body. Our feet point straight ahead and our head rests directly above our shoulders.

Imbalance comes in many forms. Here the head is tilting forward from the shoulders and the thoracic back has an exaggerated curve. The right shoulder is elevated and the hips are uneven. And, the feet do not point forward. All of these asymmetries are signs of imbalance.

the environment within our body—the sensation of hunger or thirst that grabs your attention when your body needs nutrients or hydration, the desire to gasp for air that drives you from the pool bottom during an attempt to hold your breath as long as possible. Whatever the source, stimuli trigger reactions, and those reactions require movement.

Today, the modern fetus emerges into an environment that demands less and less motion. What we do for work, play, and survival no longer fully engages our major musculoskeletal functions. From prehistoric times to about the twentieth century, the world was physically a very stimulating place for humankind. Earth was a terrestrial obstacle course, with wild animals, forest fires, towering mountains, bloodthirsty enemies, trackless deserts, and surging waters. Faced with these obstacles, our ancestors developed thousands of biomechanical and biochemical adaptations driven by environmental stimuli with one purpose—survival.

Our musculoskeletal system today is the evolutionary product of the unceasing influence of environmental stimuli. But just as that environmental stimulus was a necessity for its creation, environmental stimulus is required for its maintenance. For us, unlike our ancestors, technology and modern-day advances have significantly decreased the amount of movement required in our reactions to environmental stimuli. Our ancestors were forced to move. We can "survive" without hunting, growing crops, building shelter, finding water, or making clothes. Our ancestors could not.

Today, absent a conscious choice to react to stimuli with more movement, we can survive with a musculoskeletal system that is starved of motion. But guess what—the body adapts our musculoskeletal system to that motion-starved environment. Musculoskeletal dysfunctions are often the consequence of adaptation to our motionless life circumstances.

In the case of the musculoskeletal system, there are two

Paths to Pain Free

John Campbell, Founder, Matuse Wetsuits

John Campbell was a middle schooler when I met him; his father and I were stationed together for eighteen months in the military. He was a great athlete—playing basketball, baseball, and football—and always a fast-twitch speedster. We ended up training together intensely for ten years, as he grew to be the captain of his high school football team and went on to play football and run track at Dartmouth.

One advantage of the training was that it wasn't just about keeping the body pain free, but also about helping performance, Campbell says. Specifically, that meant he became extremely kinesthetically aware.

"You end up realizing the importance of the positioning of the hips and how that affects the alignment of the back and how if the hips and back are aligned properly, the knees and ankles and feet seem to work better," he says. "So you end up being able to move better and move more in tune with how you're supposed to function."

At five foot nine and 178 pounds, Campbell wasn't big in football terms—he played running back in high school and kick returner and cornerback in college. "I never felt undersized or undermatched," he says. "I felt that Pete's regimen always gave me a distinct advantage no matter what."

stages to pass from a normal, functional state to a pathological state of dysfunction. First, muscles that are not regularly stimulated are put on hold to atrophy until they are needed again. This is an adaptive consequence of our development in a world that previously was full of scarcity. Today, many of us enjoy access to food and water without much concern for scarcity, but that was not always the case throughout our evolution. Excess anything was a threat to survival, a drain on precious resources. The body interprets an unused muscle as wasteful, and the body is incredibly thrifty. Unused muscles steadily dwindle in size and strength, allowing the body to put the conserved resources and energy into more readily used functions.

But every now and then, even the most sedentary man, woman, or child is asked to climb stairs, run, bend over, or pick up a heavy object. Such a task requires the movement of bones by muscles. Muscles require strength to accomplish this work, and atrophied muscles simply are not up to the task. The body, driven by the certain knowledge that it must move, adapts. It hijacks surrounding muscles to do the work.

The body's brilliant ability to adapt allows us to move, but the wrong muscles are doing the work. Compensating muscles are forced to withstand a workload for which they are not designed. Think of our major movers (the big muscles designed to power movement) as large elevators rated to five thousand pounds, capable of carrying twenty-plus people up a skyscraper day in and day out without difficulty. The smaller surrounding muscles that end up picking up the slack when the major movers are not up to the task are the equivalent of a backup elevator rated to two thousand pounds. The small elevator must make at least twice as many trips or strain under a load that it is not designed to withstand to shuttle the same number of people skyward. The small elevator will not be able to withstand that demand for long, and our compensating muscles are no different.

Our musculoskeletal system can adapt by making compensating muscles stronger, but that further disrupts the delicate balance of our system. Even if our compensating muscles manage to meet this demand, the surrounding ligaments, tendons, bones, and joints are not designed to withstand that increased burden. This abnormal stress inevitably results in inefficiency, pain, and injury.

All adaptations are the result of our body desperately trying to meet our demands. Our body is the equivalent of a loyal golden retriever—deep down it would do anything to make us happy. Muscle atrophy is a response to our demand to remain

Listen to Your Body

Stimulus
the thing, event, or decision that causes us to react and move

Adaptation
the adjustment the body makes when our underlying muscle function is inadequate to achieve our desired movement

Compensation
the long-term consequence of repetitive adaptation resulting in persistent imbalance and musculoskeletal dysfunction

If we can't meet the demand of the stimulus, we adapt. That adaptation allows us to move. If we consistently rely on that adaptation to move, compensation creates persistent imbalance. Such imbalance impacts our ability to respond to subsequent stimuli, and the cycle starts anew.

stationary. Compensation is a response to our sudden demand for movement. Pain and injury are the body's last resort. When it can no longer adapt and meet our demands, when the consequences of its adaptations are causing problems that it simply cannot solve, the body asks for help. Pain is the body's voice, alerting us to a problem and asking for our help to fix it.

The Body Is a Unit

Musculoskeletal dysfunction results from imbalances in muscle strength and flexibility, which limit movement and create abnormal stress on the bones, joints, and muscles. These dysfunctions are reinforced by our movement patterns. The adaptation of our function results in disproportionate strength in compensating muscles and progressive, unaddressed weakness in less active muscles.

Just as our muscles have an incredible ability to adapt, our brain pathways also have incredible plasticity. The adaptations of the musculoskeletal system are reflected in the brain. The degree and frequency of muscle activation are reflected in our neurological pathways.

MRIs of the brain following immobilization of the forearm and hand showed decreased tissue thickness in areas of the brain responsible for movement and feeling in the immobilized extremity. Likewise, increased tissue thickness was seen in areas of the brain responsible for movement and feeling in the opposite forearm and hand, consistent with the increased activity burden created by having one arm immobilized. These changes disappear when immobilization ends.

Regular overuse causes compensating muscles to occupy a disproportionate amount of brain space compared to less active, weak muscles. This brain reorganization further reinforces dysfunctional movement patterns. Large, regularly used brain areas are like high-speed highways, connecting two points

Paths to Pain Free

Dr. Michael Lardon, Mental Performance Coach

Dr. Michael Lardon has always been into elite performance. When he was younger, he was a national champion table tennis player. In college, his lab partner was five-time Olympic gold medalist Eric Heiden. After college, his brother earned his way onto the PGA Tour.

Lardon made it his career to study elite performance—focusing on the mental aspect. His clients have included five golfers who have gone on to win major championships. In addition, he has helped many Olympic medalists and UFC world champions.

The mental side is inevitably tied to the physical side, so he often works with athletes through both issues. He was first introduced to The Egoscue Method after Jack Nicklaus publicly thanked Pete Egoscue for resurrecting his career. After integrating The Egoscue Method into his own personal life, he has referred many of his elite athlete clients to Egoscue for treatment and training. He has witnessed the success his athletes have had through the Egoscue training methods. He states that the improvements his clients have experienced with their posture and balance have had major positive effects on their careers. He says that although The Egoscue Method, which is over thirty years old, is not two thousand years old like acupuncture, it's still being used by our country's best athletes. Lardon says, "I've just seen it do a lot of good things and I've never seen it do a bad thing."

---

quickly without interruption. Underutilized, smaller areas are like dirt back roads, connecting two points in a roundabout manner, slowed by potholes and the occasional wild animal. When it comes to the brain, efficiency is the name of the game. When every second counts, you just don't bother with the back road.

The reinforcement of dysfunctional movement on the musculoskeletal and neurological level helps to explain why micro-focused therapy approaches frequently fail. The work of a weak, inactive muscle is being performed by other compensating muscles. Left unaddressed, the body will use the same reinforced movement patterns in therapy. Strengthening the weak, inactive muscle is a necessity, but too often the compensating muscles absorb the entire stimulus, leaving the weak muscle unengaged and at an even greater disadvantage.

Efforts to isolate muscles rarely work as intended, since muscles function in collaboration with one another. For example, the psoas, which is the strongest hip flexor in the body, requires collaboration from the back and abdominal muscles to function properly. Weak psoas muscles are a common cause of back pain, but attempts to strengthen the psoas are unlikely to succeed if they fail to account for the role that the back and abdominal muscles play in its function.

The musculoskeletal system is an interconnected network of unbroken muscular chains running from head to toe. This kinetic chain responds globally, with any muscle activation resonating throughout the entire musculoskeletal network. Movement, no matter how small, has a domino effect throughout the entire body. Our micro focus often fails to account for this macro ripple effect, an oversight that hinders our ability to meaningfully correct dysfunction.

The body functions as a unit. Each system is interconnected, affecting and being affected by every other system within the body.

The side effects of medications clearly illustrate this principle. A drug may cure one problem, but it will often cause another in the process (e.g., a painkiller takes away the pain but causes an upset stomach). The body does not work in a compartmentalized way. All drugs have side effects—big or small—because our interconnected nature makes isolating and affecting just one system impossible. The musculoskeletal system is no different. Isolating and affecting just one muscle, bone, or joint is impossible.

Understanding Pain: Our Perception Versus Reality

Pain as a Messenger

Pain is the body's form of high-priority communication.
Pain has one function and one function only: to alert us to danger.
Pain is the body's way of saying, "*Something* is happening that
should *not* be happening." The cure comes from eliminating or
managing that *something*. The problem boils down to identify-
ing that *something,* and when it comes to musculoskeletal pain,
we are looking in all the wrong places.

   The problem with today's approach to musculoskeletal med-

icine comes in large part from misconstruing joints as simple—
or at least as less complicated than the other major organ systems. The mechanical nature of the musculoskeletal system
seems less complex than the chemical processes of the kidneys,
the gas exchange occurring in the lungs, or the physiological
intricacies of the cardiovascular system. We fall into the false
belief that we can isolate and fix distinct parts of the musculoskeletal system without considering or influencing the body as
a whole. We become laser-focused on what hurts, and we
use sophisticated imaging and diagnostics to discover "what" is
causing our pain. We assume that the "what" is our *something*
and we stop our search. But that assumption is wrong. The
"what" is a result of our *something*. Our *something* is the "why"
that caused our "what" (and our pain) to begin with.

Think of pain as the body's built-in car alarm. Many aspects
of modern musculoskeletal medicine are akin to silencing the
car alarm with the touch of a button. The annoyance is gone,
but the alarm serves its purpose only if you also recognize the
need to look for, find, and fix the broken window that triggered
your car alarm (the "what"). Otherwise, the thief who broke
your window has an even easier time causing trouble when
he circles back around the block. But now let's consider what
happens when you fix the window but don't call the police.
The thief is your "why"—he caused the "what" that set off
your car alarm. If you don't call the police and eliminate the
thief, there is a good chance you will just end up with another
broken window.

Pain is your body's way of alerting you to an imbalance
or hiccup in your body's function. It is a signal that the abnormal
stress on your bones, joints, and muscles is causing damage.
Although it might feel like someone is incessantly yelling
at you, at its core, pain in simply trying to talk to you. Your job
is to listen. My job is to show you how to translate pain's
message.

Common Pain Misconceptions

You no doubt consider yourself quite familiar with pain, and you likely have a lot of words to describe the pain you experience—many of which I can't print in this book. Although screaming profanities can disperse some anger and frustration, those words do nothing to help you understand pain.

Translating pain's message requires understanding pain's language. Unfortunately, we all too often face a huge linguistic barrier when it comes to pain. Many of our common perceptions about pain are not just wrong—they are holding us back when it comes to fixing our pain problem.

Movement as a Villain

I often hear people say they are afraid to move. Many of these individuals are reluctant to move out of fear that movement will worsen their pain. If hamstring pain follows a run, or back pain follows a bike ride, the easiest solution is not to run or bike, right? Perhaps, but concluding that movement is the cause of pain confuses correlation with causation. While movement is frequently correlated with pain, this casual conclusion does not consider a key question: Why is movement hurting me?

A year ago, you could run without hamstring pain. A year ago, the act of running wasn't causing pain. Today, you get hamstring pain only on your left side. Today, the act of running is not causing pain in your right hamstring.

Movement cannot be our villain because it doesn't account for these differences. There must be some difference on your left side that is not present on your right side and was not present last year. That difference is musculoskeletal function. The problem is not movement. The problem is *how* you are moving. Imbalance in muscle strength and flexibility changes how we move and over-stresses certain areas of our musculo-skeletal system, creating pain and injury.

Reality Check: Pain is a consequence of how we are moving. Movement is not the problem. We are at an all-time high of feeling at an all-time low because we are moving less when we need to be moving more.

Pain as a Symptom of Getting Old or Wearing Out

Too often we assume that our pain is a symptom of the inevitable wear and tear that comes with getting old. After all, pain is more common as we age, and pain is often correlated with nasty X-rays and MRIs that show damage to our joints and surrounding tissues. But there are far too many exceptions to these correlations to blame age and musculoskeletal wear and tear for our pain problem.

Ed Whitlock ran the Toronto Marathon in 2016 at the age of eighty-five. He completed the 26.2-mile course in three hours and fifty-six minutes, becoming the oldest person to finish the distance in under four hours. The feat impressed even the most knowledgeable sport performance scientists. Testing showed that Whitlock retained an exceptional amount of muscle mass despite his advancing age.

Motor units—a neuron and its surrounding muscle fibers—are the smallest functional entity of our muscles. Motor units typically decline with age, correlating with declines in muscle mass and strength. An average, healthy twenty-year-old will have about 160 motor units in the anterior tibialis, the muscle that runs along the front of the shin and helps to pick up the toes when walking or running. By age eighty, that number of

Paths to Pain Free

Loren Lahav, International Speaker

I met Loren Lahav almost three decades ago at a Tony Robbins event. She still remembers what I said to her when I saw her: "You have natural turnout of the hips, like a ballerina. And you'll never be able to carry a baby full term—your hip flexors are too weak."

I didn't know it at the time, but she had had two miscarriages.

She started going to our clinic, and doesn't have the turnout anymore. She got pregnant a couple years later (and now has three kids, ages twenty-four, twenty, and thirteen).

Plus, she has no back pain—even though she's fifty-five, travels two hundred days a year, and wears four-inch heels when she's onstage for her speaking engagements. Every time she gets off the plane, her E-cises are one of the first things she does.

"I can go all day and have never been in pain. It changed my life. I live it," she says. "It's part of who I am. What I'm most proud of is that my kids have seen me do it consistently and do the E-cises as well."

---

motor units typically declines to 60. Whitlock came in close to 100.

Our body does not measure birthdays, but it does measure muscle strength and muscle function. The problem is getting weak, not old.

Imaging studies provide a lot of detailed information about our musculoskeletal system, but the findings on X-rays, CT scans, and MRIs all too often do not correlate with pain. Osteoarthritis is frequently referred to as "wear and tear" arthritis. Arthritis is easily seen on X-rays. But the presence of arthritis on X-rays is an extremely poor predictor of pain. Two individuals can have the same severity of arthritis on X-rays and have drastically different experiences with pain. One might suffer debilitating agony while the other does not experience even mild pain. In fact, 80 percent of adults over the age of 55 have signs of arthritis on knee X-rays. Thankfully, not nearly that many people actually experience knee pain. The bottom line: Pain does not correlate with the presence of osteoarthritis on X-rays.

MRI findings in the lower back are similar. In a study of individuals without any complaints of back pain, 37 percent of twenty-year-old individuals had signs of disc degeneration on their MRIs. That percentage increased to 96 percent in the pain-free eighty-year-old population. Traditional signs of musculo-skeletal wear and tear on all types of imaging fail to consistently correspond with pain.

Reality Check: Pain is not the result of growing old or wearing out. Age and imaging abnormalities fail to adequately account for our current pain epidemic.

Pain as a Sign of Fragility

Pain, particularly in the absence of adequate relief and predictability, often leaves us feeling fragile. When we are faced with an inability to reliably relieve our pain and an inability to predict when or where we will hurt, it is easy to feel frustrated. This lack of understanding makes us feel disconnected from our body. It becomes easy to criticize our musculoskeletal system as weak or inferior and to accept that fragility as fact.

My hope is that by this point you know that nothing could be further from the truth. The body is not weak, inferior, or fragile. It is perfectly designed and incredibly versatile. It responds to stimuli with such adaptive prowess that we can move even under the most compromised conditions.

Our body responds to pain just like any other environmental stimulus. When we experience pain with a movement, our mus-culoskeletal system adapts its response. When we move and feel

Paths to Pain Free

Ollie, College Soccer Player

Ollie had been sprinting when he felt a pain that he thought was a groin pull. He would rest and feel better but the pain would come back the next time he tried to play soccer. He didn't want to be hampered during the season. He was at an important moment in his college recruiting process and was eager to get back to playing.

He started doing Egoscue E-cises to realign himself and fix his posture, and within a few weeks he felt ready to get back at it. He hasn't had a problem ever since. And he still does Cats and Dogs (page 85) before practices and games.

"I think it made me play better as a result," says Ollie, who went on to land a scholarship to play at a dream school.

---

pain, the body inhibits further activity in the muscles responsible for producing the painful movement. Likewise, activity is increased in muscles that would normally resist the painful movement. The body senses pain and alters muscle activation to try and prevent repeating the same painful movement over again.

Similarly, the brain modifies its activity and signaling pathways if acute pain lingers and becomes a chronic problem. MRIs performed during acute episodes of back pain showed activation of brain areas responsible for processing painful stimuli. Subsequent MRIs performed on the same individuals who continued to experience back pain for two-plus years yielded vastly different results. Areas of the brain responsible for the control of emotion showed large increases in activity. Other areas responsible for motivation and inhibition of our perception of pain showed decreased activity. These changes correlate with the complaints of fatigue, hypersensitivity, and emotional volatility seen with chronic pain but generally absent with acute pain.

The changes seen in muscle activation and brain activity are transient. They are generally seen in response to pain, and are reversible when the pain resolves.

Unrelenting pain changes our neurological wiring, creating feelings of fragility, fatigue, and hopelessness. Those feelings increase the likelihood that we make negative self-judgments, but pain is not a sign that any of those self-judgments are true.

Reality Check: *Feelings of fragility and weakness are frequently caused by pain, but pain is not a sign that the body is fragile, weak, or inferior. Our ability to move even in the face of compromised musculoskeletal function is a testament to our resilience and strength.*

Three Surprising Things That Might Help Your Pain

Patience: Today's world moves at hyperspeed. Information is available with the click of a button. Overnight shipping will place your latest purchase at your fingertips within twenty-four hours. Uber will pick you up and take you anywhere with five minutes' notice. Emergency rooms and urgent care centers make access to medical care instant. These are wonderful conveniences, but our expectations have evolved to match our environment, and we expect instant results. The body does not work on modern society's timeline. It often takes a lot of time to develop the imbalances and weakness that ultimately result in pain. Temporary relief might be achievable with a pill or a few exercises. But just as it took months or even years to develop the imbalances that ultimately resulted in pain, long-lasting results require time and consistency.

Jack Miller, CEO, Pacific College of Health and Science (Formerly Pacific College of Oriental Medicine)

Jack Miller developed back pain from his years of surfing and competing as an amateur race car driver.

A mutual friend reminded him of The Egoscue Method, and he started doing "menus," programs of Egoscue exercises, to relieve the pain. "I found it to be really effective and supportive of other therapies," he says. And he's now been doing it for thirteen years.

Miller added Egoscue as part of the elective curriculum at Pacific College, and one of the reasons Miller likes it so much is that you can make major improvements in a short amount of time. You can start with ten minutes a day max and work from there. And it creates a virtuous cycle—"If ten minutes is good, I'll see how fifteen feels, or maybe I'll do ten in the morning and ten in the afternoon," he says.

"It's really about empowering patients to help themselves," he says.

Giving Up the Desire for Certainty: An emergency room physician recently told me that one of the most surprising things she had learned was that for many people a diagnosis, even a bad diagnosis, was often better received than no diagnosis. Even when no diagnosis was prefaced with the good news that a patient's CT scan showed no signs of any life-threatening ailments, frustration was more common than relief when the question of what caused their pain was left unanswered. We simply despise uncertainty. Certainty is powerful because it removes our sense of personal responsibility. If we have a definitive diagnosis, there is a preestablished treatment plan that *should* work. If that treatment is not successful, it is the result of a shortcoming on the part of the medical establishment. Remember, shy of acute trauma, most musculoskeletal pain is triggered by imbalance that results from insufficient, repetitive movement patterns. In the musculoskeletal world, certainty comes as a diagnosis provided by X-rays, MRIs, and CT scans. Too often, we anchor on that certainty and entirely overlook the imbalance that caused our diagnosis to begin with.

Letting Go of "Fix Me": When it comes to pain, there is a huge difference in outcomes between patients who choose the driver's seat and those who elect to sit passively in the passenger seat. "Please fix me" is a far too common plea of pain patients to medical professionals. While it is completely normal to wish that pain could simply be taken away, everything we have learned about the successful treatment of chronic pain suggests that that is just not the way things work. Whether through daily exercise, medication, or routine participation in activities that bring joy, patients who actively engage in their pain treatment have better outcomes. By moving to the driver's seat, you are accepting an active role in your treatment and accepting some responsibility for the control of your symptoms. There is unquestionably a place for medical expertise, but no one will ever be as much of an expert on you as you.

5

The Egoscue Method: A Life in Balance

Life is like riding a bicycle. To keep your balance, you must keep moving.

—Albert Einstein

If you have ever chased success, you have most likely learned the importance of balance. The world's most successful businessmen and CEOs are regularly quoted preaching the importance of balance to their success. Athletes are constantly trying to balance the impact of hard training with the necessity of recovery for growth and improvement. Physicians balance the benefits of medical interventions with adverse side effects. When balance shifts too far to one side of the scale, problems ensue.

The body is no different. It wants and needs balance. Problems ensue when balance is lost.

One of the major challenges faced in our modern musculoskeletal pain epidemic is how numb we have become to the inner workings of our body. We are becoming less and less capable of recognizing and correcting musculoskeletal imbalance before it causes problems because we are becoming less and less aware of what balance *feels* like.

When I speak to groups, I often poll the audience to see who is experiencing pain. Maybe fifteen years ago, a fraction of the group would raise their hands to show that they did not feel so great. About ten years ago, just about everyone raised their hands. Now almost nobody raises their hands. On the surface, fewer people acknowledging pain seems like a positive. But what I have found is that the opposite is true: almost everyone feels lousy. Small aches and pains have become so much the norm that these discomforts no longer even register on our kinesthetic radar.

Being numb is not a sign of good health. Ignorance may be bliss when it comes to the mysteries of auto repair, computers, and landscaping, but for our musculoskeletal system, ignorance is pain.

Numbness is possible only when we become disconnected from our kinesthetic sense—the ability to accurately *feel* the positions and movements of our bones, joints, and muscles. Kinesthetic sense allows us to detect when we are bearing 70 percent of our weight on one side of our body. It allows us to sense when our leg stops straightening out during our gait. It allows us to recognize when one shoulder has far greater mobility than the other. If pain is the body's form of an emergency alert system, kinesthetic sense is akin to the weather forecast that alerts us to the impending hurricane before it makes landfall. Kinesthetic sense allows us to recognize dysfunction and musculoskeletal stress before the body reaches for its last resort—pain.

Paths to Pain Free

Simon Reed, VP Sales, Insurance Company

Simon Reed had always been an active guy. He played soccer and did martial arts. But after college, he got a desk job and spent most of his days seated. He went from limber to sedentary—doing all the things you do when you get married, have children, purchase a home, and own a business.

"I had a big old ugly chair in my insurance office, and one day I carried it out to the dumpster. It was raining, so there was a mud patch between the dumpster and the blacktop. So I just heaved the chair twelve feet and lobbed it into the dumpster," he says.

He didn't think anything of it at the moment, but he felt *something*.

By the time he got back to his office a few hundred yards away, he knew something was wrong. That sent him on a downward spiral.

He had a herniated disc—and couldn't do a thing. Couldn't stand. Couldn't sit. Couldn't bend to tie his shoelaces.

Reed tried everything—medications, physical therapy. Eventually doctors wanted to get more aggressive—with the eventual outcome being the removal of the disc and fusing of the spine. He was limited in what he could do, which even caused marital tension because of his inability to move.

Through a mutual connection with his sister, Reed found Egoscue. Reed overnighted a video of himself walking and was given a series of E-cises to do. He did them religiously. He was realigning everything.

Between days 55 and 60 of doing his menu every day, the pain went away—and never came back.

A couple weeks later, he went out to do some yardwork (which he had not been able to do since the injury). He did it for about eight hours, and his neighbor told him he was going to feel it the next day. He didn't. Just a couple weeks removed from not being able to move, he was out there working hard, operating a chainsaw and clearing debris. To this day, he rarely misses doing a day of E-cises (and he's been doing them for twenty-two years) because he knows that it saved his back—and his movement.

"To say that it works is an understatement," he says. "I'm living it."

Without kinesthetic sense, there is no objective standard for what dysfunctional joints and muscles feel like—until they start to hurt.

What We Do

The Egoscue Method fills the stimulus gap created by our sedentary environment with a unique program of exercises known as E-cises that target muscles undergoing inadequate or improper motion. These E-cises amount to muscle and joint tutorials—reteaching the muscles what to do and how to do it.

E-cises serve two purposes. The first should seem relatively straightforward to you at this point. E-cises restore the critical balance of the kinetic chain and allow muscles to relearn their correct role in movement. The dynamic tension between muscle groups is reestablished, improving the vertical alignment of our joints to maximize musculoskeletal function. A functional musculoskeletal system not only is efficient but also minimizes the stress on bones, joints, and muscles most commonly responsible for musculoskeletal pain.

The second purpose of E-cises is less obvious but no less important. Many of our clients arrive with pain as their only reference point to their body. Their attention is riveted to the spot that hurts, and they have become numb to their kinesthetic sense. Kinesthetic sense provides the standard for what a functional musculoskeletal system *feels* like. E-cises supply that missing standard—allowing clients to see and ultimately feel musculoskeletal function. That awakening restores our innate kinesthetic sense, allowing the body to detect imbalance and dysfunction in the absence of pain.

In short, The Egoscue Method does two things: (1) restores the balance of the musculoskeletal system and (2) reestablishes the body's innate early-detection system to sense changes in that balance.

Paths to Pain Free

Laurie-Ann Weis

When she was eighteen, Laurie-Ann Weis was in a serious car accident that left her with severe back pain. "It destroyed my life as I knew it," she says. "I struggled for years in and out of therapy. Nothing worked. Everyone who touched me made me worse. I went from a very promising life to a very difficult life."

She couldn't sit comfortably in cars and had to lie down in the back seat. She couldn't stand and could sit for only twenty minutes. She was bedridden for most of her young adult life.

Doctors tried everything—medications, physical therapy, yoga. She had a failed spinal surgery, which made her hip move out of alignment, causing her severe pain.

One day, an endocrinologist whom she had been seeing told her, "I know this isn't my business and I know this isn't my field, but I wanted to tell you about another patient I had who went to a place called Egoscue. I have seen miracles with this man, and I think this is what you need."

We started working together, and Laurie-Ann started to have moments when she didn't experience any pain as she learned how to realign her body. She felt changes immediately, though it took time to retrain the muscle memory.

That was thirty-four years ago. Today, she does the program at least six days a week to keep her body aligned for a pain-free, fulfilling life. She does selected E-cises spontaneously to help her get out of a little pain or soreness she feels as needed. But the chronic debilitating pain? It's gone.

"I started with the basics, and little by little, the pain and weakness slowly went away," she says. "I had to learn to realign my whole body and to have hope again. He gave me a life—a pain-free life."

Less pain is what brought you here, but my hope is that by now you have recognized the key role that movement plays not only in our musculoskeletal system but in our physical and mental health. The Egoscue Method will help you get out of pain and restore your musculoskeletal system to a balanced state where movement is possible and joyful. The choice to move more—well, that is all yours.

Where to Start

THE QUESTION YOU MUST ASK

When I talk to someone with pain, the first question I hear is this: How can I fix it? That's a good question (and that's what this book is about), but that's not what will propel you forward to help yourself.

The better question is: What can't you do now that you would like to do?

What is your pain preventing you from doing? What part of life are you not engaging in that you want to? What used to bring you happiness, satisfaction, and joy that you can no longer do? Gardening, playing basketball or tennis, traveling? Whatever your answer, that can become the driver of everything you do from here on out.

The potential of returning to the life you want will be the driving force that helps you persevere through roadblocks and make the changes necessary to help yourself. As we discuss posture, movement, and ways to improve those things, I want you to remember your *why*. That untapped potential should remain a central part of your journey toward self-reliance.

Your actions will be propelled by your inspiration.

Case in point: When videogames started to boom, I saw a lot of parents who became concerned that their kids were sitting all the time. They complained that their kids were start-

Paths to Pain Free

Steven Shea, Film Producer

Steven Shea was picked to be on the YouTube reality series *Becoming Pain Free* because he had one of the worst alignments I have seen—probably from years editing at a desk. He was also having a lot of back pain and achiness, and he had a hard time picking up his son. In addition, he had a lot of wrist pain and hadn't gotten any results from different things he had tried.

In the first E-cise he did, he started cramping up—and that was just standing against a wall. But he stuck with it. After eight weeks, there were drastic differences in his spine—and he felt better all over.

"One of the things that stuck with me was this idea of side effects. Your body is connected, and everything needs to run correctly to work right," he says. "The wrist pain was a side effect of my back not being straight. When we found the problem, the side effect went away."

He now does his E-cises to help fend off the temporary pain he may feel from working, and he has felt his overall chronic pain lessen.

"I even grew an inch because my back straightened out," he says.

---

ing to look like Quasimodo. As a result of sitting for hours on end, day after day, glued to a videogame on a TV screen, their posture was going to hell. These parents noticed the change and grew concerned by the unhealthy appearance of their children.

But did the kids care? Their friends all looked the same way, and they liked playing their videogames. They were not at all concerned that their spine was more curved than a coiled snake.

You know what worked? I asked them some questions: What's your favorite game? What's your best score?

Then I told them that they could improve their score by improving the way that their bodies functioned. That potential for improvement appealed to them; it inspired action.

A coiled spine did not resonate with them, but they sure as hell cared about how their body worked when put into the context of a videogame. The kids readily completed their posture exercises and went back to gaming ready to post new high scores.

Part of your evolution in becoming pain free will include reframing your pain problem. Focusing on what you want out of life is the first positive step toward empowering your body to help you get there.

The Twenty-Second Self-Test

Take off your shoes and stand up. Close your eyes. Take note of where you feel the weight is distributed in your feet. Compare how that weight feels on your left foot versus your right foot. If you are like most modern humans, it will not be long before you notice differences. You might feel much less pressure in one foot compared to the other. You might feel weight concentrated on the front of your left foot but on the back of your right. You might notice that all your weight runs along the outside of your right foot versus a balanced distribution across your left. All of these differences are signs of imbalance.

Remember our discussion about our design. We are intended to be symmetric bipeds. The right side of our musculoskeletal system should identically mirror the left side. If you are noticing differences in your weight distribution from side to side, you are noticing asymmetries. The Egoscue Method will help you correct those imbalances. If you have pain now, improving those imbalances will alleviate your symptoms. If you don't have pain, improving those imbalances will prevent the inevitable progression of dysfunction, helping you avoid pain and injury in the future.

Steps to Moving Forward

Reconnect with your resilience

Make it your mission to move more (whether it's with formal exercise or just getting off the couch)

Perform your self-test to see if you are imbalanced

Start your menu of E-cises (after learning more about them here) and begin treating the source of your pain

Learn more about your imbalance and start using E-cises to treat the source of your pain.

The next several chapters explore individual joints and common causes of dysfunction and pain unique to these joints. The menus within each chapter will serve as the program of E-cises that you will follow to become pain free. Flip to the section that highlights where you feel pain and follow the menu. In doing so, you will teach your muscles to correct the imbalances causing your pain.

Everyone will react differently. Some may experience complete relief after one menu. Others may notice smaller amounts of relief immediately with steady improvement from subsequent menus. Others might feel relief in one area but start experiencing pain somewhere new. No need to panic—simply jump to that section of the book and follow the menu designed to address your new pain.

The most important thing to remember is that your body did not get to a state of chronic pain overnight. It took months—even years—of repetitive dysfunction and imbalance. E-cises provide a repetitive stimulus through which our bodies can unlearn those dysfunctions and relearn functional, balanced movement patterns. "One and done" might relieve your pain for a time, but long-lasting relief comes from consistent, positive stimulus and the power of the body to adapt to that stimulus.

Assessing Balance

Assessing balance can be challenging. CEOs and corporate executives often score themselves on seven elements they consider crucial to a balanced life—physical health, family, social life, business, financial health, civic engagement, and spiritual health. Athletes monitor their resting heart rate, weight, and fatigue levels to gauge the balance of their current training regimen.

In medicine, balance is often assessed with tests that measure invisible parameters within the body. Nutrition can be assessed with measurements of cholesterol, blood glucose, and fat levels. Hydration can be assessed with measurements of kidney function and electrolytes. The musculoskeletal system offers a unique advantage because we can see and feel the balance of our muscles, bones, and joints without fancy tests or needlesticks.

6

Feet and Ankles: Our Musculoskeletal Sole

We have a love-hate relationship with our feet. No other single body part generates anything close to the billions of dollars we spend to keep our feet comfortable, sexy, and hip. Yet we simultaneously expect our feet to toil like peasants and never complain. But more often than we would like, pain overpowers the desired culture-of-silence status quo.

The feet are designed to support the weight of our entire body. Our fully erect posture—a feature we share with no other mammal—rests entirely on our two feet. The average human used to take ten thousand steps per day, enough to circle the

Fibula
Tibia

Talus
(ankle bone)

Calcaneus
(heel bone)

The ankle joint consists of the fibula, tibia, and talus. The bottom bone of the ankle, the talus, connects directly to the bones of the foot.

globe four times over an average life span. Today, that number is closer to three thousand (a glaring example of just how far we have fallen from motion-filled grace). Regardless, the feet bear the entirety of our weight throughout every step of that journey.

Our feet may be small, but what they lack in size they more than make up for in structural might. In a typical day, our feet withstand several hundred tons of cumulative force. The bones of the feet account for a quarter of all the bones in the body, and the sole of the foot has more than two hundred thousand nerve endings. Our feet are—quite literally—designed for the long haul.

The Great Shoe Hijack

Ever wonder what's behind all the shoes claiming to correct overpronation? Supination and pronation are normal movements of the ankle and foot that help to navigate the divide between the flexibility needed for shock absorption and balance and the rigidity necessary for stability and forward propulsion in gait. When the arches of the foot are compromised, so too is the body's ability to deal with the nuances of surface variation, foot strike, and weight distribution. The muscles of the lower leg use supination and pronation as a substitute for those lost functions.

Overpronation increases our ability to accommodate for uneven terrain and assists with maintaining balance. But hijacking this function to facilitate balance compromises shock absorption and forward propulsion. Likewise, oversupination provides additional foot rigidity and stability, but this compromises shock absorption and balance.

The bones of the feet form three distinct arches that give the foot the mobility necessary for balance and gait. We are not born with this characteristic arch structure in our feet. Babies are born with a pad of fat where the arches will ultimately come to reside. The bony arches develop as a consequence of our ongoing demand to stand and walk upright. Supported by ligaments, tendons, and muscles, these arches are designed to act as a spring, buffering force and increasing the efficiency of two-legged ambulation.

Like other musculoskeletal functions, the balanced state of the foot arches can be maintained only through movement.

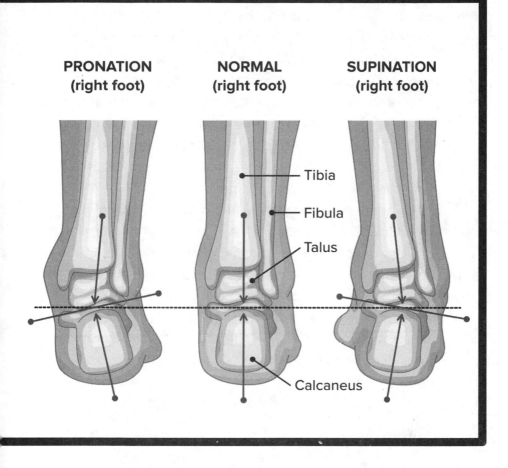

PRONATION
(right foot)

NORMAL
(right foot)

SUPINATION
(right foot)

Tibia

Fibula

Talus

Calcaneus

When the feet point straight ahead, walking gait provides a more than adequate stimulus to maintain the muscle function necessary for arch structure. Inadequate or imbalanced stimulus triggers changes in our arches. Such change alters the energy efficiency of our gait and disrupts the distribution of shock generated during movement.

The ankle joint works closely with the foot to coordinate our interaction with the ground. The ankle is the junction where the bones of the lower leg (the tibia and fibula) meet the foot. Ankles often get a bad rap as being weak and injury prone. In reality, the ankle has a built-in private security team composed of the muscles, ligaments, and tendons that surround and support the joint. Our all-terrain, mobile nature is made possible by the combined movements of the ankle and foot joints. That mobility requires support, and the foot and ankle have more than one hundred ligaments that help to stabilize movement. Combined with the strength of the surrounding muscles, that is a hearty first line of defense. But most people have muscle weakness and imbalance that infiltrate these built-in defenses, increasing the likelihood of injury and pain.

The ankle acts as the linchpin that keeps our body upright and balanced over our foot. It processes input about terrain variability, foot position, and the ongoing movements of our legs, torso, and upper body to make split-second adjustments that keep us stable and vertical. If you think of the foot as an anchor and the rest of your body as a ship, the ankle serves as the chain that connects the two. Often when the ship and anchor are at odds, it is the chain that balances those opposing forces and keeps everything connected. But the chain is also usually the first thing to break if those opposing forces cannot be balanced.

Power in Numbers

The muscles of our foot and lower leg work as a team to adjust foot strike and accommodate for uneven terrain while simultaneously absorbing the force of impact, distributing weight, and maintaining balance. During foot strike, our foot needs the flexibility to adjust to uneven terrain. Later in the gait cycle, our foot needs to be rigid to propel the weight of our body forward.

The foot functions much like the four tires of a car. The two front wheels are located on either side of the ball of the foot, and the rear tires sit on either side of the heel. Cars drive best when they are aligned and the tires are balanced. The foot is

Arches: High or Flat?

Flat arches place the entirety of the sole in contact with the ground and reduce the ability of the foot to absorb force (think driving around on flat tires). High arches leave less surface area in contact with the ground, disproportionately concentrating impact at the front and rear of the foot (think driving around on four small spare tires). Changes in force distribution and absorption increase the likelihood of injury. Adults with flat feet have a significantly greater likelihood of reporting back and lower limb pain. Individuals with high arches are at greater risk of bony injuries in the foot and plantar fasciitis (inflammation of the fascia running along the bottom of the foot).

Ankle Sprains

The ankle joint is more stable in dorsiflexion (toes pulled up) and less stable in plantarflexion (toes pointed). This is because the bottom bone of the ankle is wider toward the front of the foot. This is why most ankle sprains occur when we are first putting down our foot or getting ready to push off the ground.

no different. The sole's high concentration of sensory neurons allows for the detection of subtle changes in the terrain beneath the foot. The muscles of our foot work in combination with our arches to react to that information, making minute adjustments to keep pressure balanced across all four of our tires.

Without a functional arch, the delicate balance of foot and ankle function quickly falls out of alignment. Our foot's ability to evenly distribute weight and absorb shock becomes compromised. Certain tires suffer more wear and tear than would be necessary if all four tires were carrying equal weight. But the damage of unbalanced tires does not stop with tire tread. Brakes also wear more quickly with misaligned tires. Fuel efficiency is decreased.

Without the shock-absorbing capacity of the arches, the foot's contact with the ground sends impact waves right up the bones of the lower leg to the knee, hip, and beyond. Similarly, as the bony structure of the arch changes, weight distribution falls increasingly to the muscles of the foot and lower leg. As these muscles are increasingly overworked with the responsibilities of weight distribution, the inherent flexibility of the foot is impaired, forcing the body to find new ways to provide the mobility necessary for gait.

The perfect partnership between our foot, ankle, and the surrounding muscles slowly falls apart. The calf, upper leg, and lower back must take over the job of orchestrating load distribution, absorbing shock, and appropriately adjusting to the ever-changing surface beneath our feet. These larger muscles are simply unsuited for such intricate work. As the body adapts, it sacrifices the nuances of complex foot function for the crude necessities needed to keep our body on its feet and moving forward.

These adaptations also compromise the stability of the foot and ankle, the platform upon which the entire body is anchored. And they create abnormal strain on the muscles, bones, and joints, ultimately resulting in injury and pain.

Bye Bye, Bunions

Bunion is a general term used to describe a deformity of the first metatarsal joint (the big joint at the base of the first toe). Most commonly, abnormal foot mechanics distort the alignment of the joint. As the bones shift out of alignment, a visible bump results along the inside of the foot. Over time, those same imbalanced mechanics pull the bones of the first toe farther and farther out of position. Eventually, the body starts to form a protective callus to buffer the increased friction of the misaligned bones. Correct the foot's balance and mechanics and the bones will move back into alignment, alleviating pain and deformity alike.

**NORMAL
(left foot)**

**BUNION
(right foot)**

A good mechanic will see unequal tire and brake wear and immediately recommend that you get an alignment. Replacing worn tires and brakes will do little good if you continue to drive around out of balance. The body is no different. We feel foot and ankle pain and rest to allow our injuries to subside. But often the same injury recurs, or a new issue arises. We replace the worn tires but skip the alignment. Alignment and long-lasting pain relief go hand in hand—we cannot have the former without the latter. And when it comes to upright movement, the feet and ankles are quite literally our one and only hope for a balanced foundation.

Plantar Fasciitis

The plantar fascia is a long band of fibrous connective tissue along the bottom of the foot that runs from the heel to the toes. It plays an important role in gait. When the mechanics of the

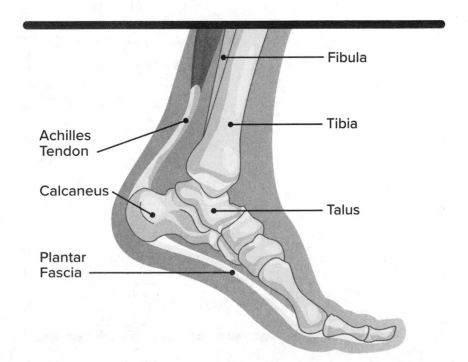

The Shoe Test

One easy way to assess your musculoskeletal balance is to look at the bottom of an old pair of shoes. Are the soles of your shoes evenly worn? Is more tread absent from the outside edge of one sole versus the other? Is the heel of one shoe more worn than the other? Odds are the soles of your shoes are not symmetrically worn. All those asymmetries mirror imbalance within your musculoskeletal system. Fun fact: You can use the same trick to monitor your progress. Just make sure you start with a fresh pair of shoes!

foot and ankle are balanced, the plantar fascia acts like an elastic band that helps generate the force necessary for forward propulsion and reduces the work required from our muscles. When our muscles fall out of balance and our joints operate with compromised mobility, the plantar fascia's ability to generate force through its elastic recoil becomes compromised, and our gait becomes less efficient. Surrounding muscles are asked to do more work to make up for this lost energy, opening the door for overuse and injury.

The plantar fascia also plays a key role in supporting and stabilizing the arch of the foot. If the muscles of the foot aren't up to the task of supporting the arch, the plantar fascia is often asked to pick up the slack. Similarly, tight calf muscles and restricted ankle mobility can increase the amount of stress the plantar fascia is asked to withstand. Either can result in the plantar fascia being overworked, which ultimately results in inflammation and pain.

Heel spurs are bony growths that can be seen on X-rays, typically along the edge of the calcaneus where the plantar fascia attaches to the heel bone. Although these bony outcroppings might seem like culprits for plantar fascia pain, generally that's not the case. Approximately one in every ten people will have heel spurs, but only one in every twenty of those individuals will experience heel pain. Heel spurs typically form as the result of plantar fasciitis; it's the body's protective mechanism to help strengthen the overworked and angry plantar fascia. Heel spurs are generally the result of plantar fasciitis, not the cause.

Unsurprisingly, the key to an energy-efficient, injury-free gait is a balanced musculoskeletal system. Special shoes, orthotics, and rest can all play a role in helping to mediate the pain, but none address the alignment issues that created the problem to begin with.

Our Achilles Heel

The Achilles tendon got a bad rap thanks to Achilles' ambitious mother, who, according to legend, dipped her infant son in the magical waters of the river Styx to make him immortal. But the greatest of all the ancient Greek warriors had one small vulnerability: the heel of the foot by which his mother held him for his mythical baptism. It remained dry and unprotected. In the last days of the Trojan War, a spear hit that one spot, with the help of the god Apollo, and killed Achilles at the gates of Troy.

Anyone who has experienced pain or injury to the Achilles tendon knows that this legend is more than just myth. Narrow in diameter and unprotected by bone or muscle mass, the Achilles rests in a vulnerable position. But what it lacks in armor, it more than makes up for in structural might. In fact, it is the largest and strongest tendon in the body. When we walk or run, the force necessary to heave our entire weight off the ground and move us forward gets transmitted through the Achilles tendon. But the

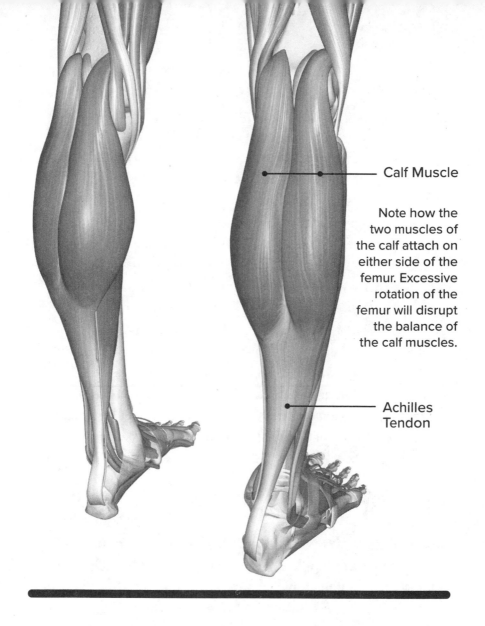

Calf Muscle

Note how the two muscles of the calf attach on either side of the femur. Excessive rotation of the femur will disrupt the balance of the calf muscles.

Achilles Tendon

demand for such strength makes the tendon particularly vulner-able to imbalance and dysfunction.

The Achilles anchors the two calf muscles to the foot. The larger calf muscle runs the length of the lower leg and splits into two tendons that attach to either side of the femur. Any knee misalignment will disrupt the dynamic tension and interac-tion of the tendons. Any lingering rotation of the femur will leave the calf tendons imbalanced, with one half of the muscle over-stretched and the opposite half extra tight. The Achilles tendon, instead of delivering a taut, smooth contraction, starts to twist and twang. And it is not designed to twist and twang.

The tendon's contractile force is such that it is capable of suddenly moving a load that is many times the weight of the body. That same strength, when turned against itself, is extremely damaging. Imbalance between the Achilles and its opposing tendons on either side of the femur produces constant friction in the fibers of the Achilles. Small tears from this friction can predispose the tendon to a complete rupture. Chronic friction can result in calcification of the tendon, worsening pain and further weakening the already compromised structure.

All sorts of special techniques have been devised to protect the Achilles, including special warm-ups, stretching, and extra-supportive footwear, but the best precaution of all is also preventative. Eliminating musculoskeletal dysfunction and imbalance is the most protective step one can take toward safeguarding our Achilles heel.

Shin Splints

Shin splints result when the tibia, the weight-bearing bone of the lower leg, and the muscles that surround it become inflamed and painful. Small microtears in the muscles, the tendons, and the outer layer of the bone result in an unrelenting dull ache typically along the front of the lower leg. Most consider this an overuse injury, but I find that label is misleading. Sure, the tissues break down and result in pain when the rate of microtrauma exceeds the rate of repair. But—and it's a *big* but—balance matters. When the body is balanced, the muscles along the shin evenly distribute work and stress. When balanced motion disappears, that work and stress become hyper-concentrated in particular areas of the muscle, tendon, and

Leg Cramps

If you develop leg cramps after starting E-cises, it's most likely a reaction to having the muscles do work that they are unaccustomed to doing. Lower leg cramps can also be caused by dehydration and electrolyte imbalances. If you routinely get foot or calf cramps, especially at night, drink more water. And lots of it. Bananas can also be a helpful source of electrolytes that can calm cramping muscles.

bone while other areas take a sabbatical. Those overworked areas can't do the work of the entire team for long without consequence. Correcting foot strike and coordinating the movements of the hip, knee, and ankle are the best strategy for healing (and preventing) this disordered disparity.

The Menu for Feet

Sitting Heel Raises with Block.......... 71

Short Foot.. 72

Static Back....................................... 73

Frog... 74

Foot Circles and Point Flexes 75

Calf/Hamstring Stretch.................... 76

Static Extension............................... 77

Air Bench... 78

Sitting Heel Raises with Block

KNOW IT: Helps to coordinate movement of the entire lower extremity.

DO IT: Sit on the edge of a chair or bench, and arch your lower back by rolling your hips forward. Place a pillow or foam block between your knees and gently squeeze the block. Your toes should remain pointed straight ahead and your big toe should remain the center point of contact with the floor throughout the motion. Raise your heels. Don't push off your toes; instead, use your hip flexor muscles (imagine your toes are resting on eggshells to keep them relaxed).

OWN IT: Do three sets of ten repetitions.

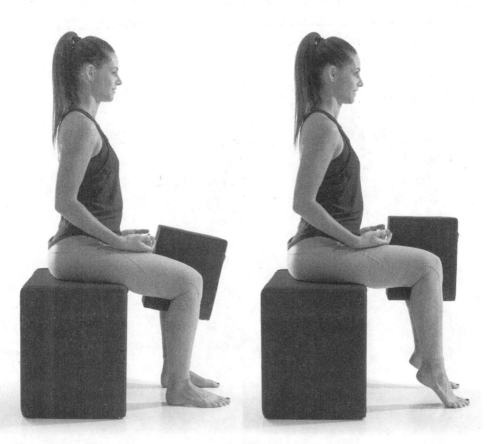

Short Foot

KNOW IT: Mimics proper foot and ankle movement during gait and starts to take away compensations in the load joints.

DO IT: Stand with your feet hip-width apart. Bring your right foot forward so that your right heel is in line with the toes of the left foot. Make sure both feet are pointing absolutely straight, and make sure your weight is evenly distributed in both feet. Bend your knees. In this position, lift the toes of the right foot up off the floor. Try to spread your toes apart as you pull them off the floor. Do not let the ball of the foot lift off the floor, lift only the toes. Next, press the toes into the floor without lifting the heel. Try to keep your toes elongated as you push down into the floor (don't curl your toes!). The arch of your foot will produce this motion, and you will feel the arch push upward when done correctly. Repeat on the other side, with the left foot in front.

OWN IT: Do three sets of ten repetitions on each side.

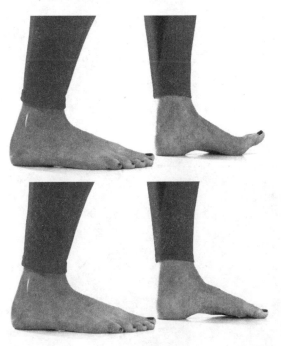

Static Back

KNOW IT: Settles your hips and back, releasing the compensating muscles that interfere with balance and functional movement.

DO IT: Lie on your back with both legs bent at right angles on a chair or block. Your hips should also be at ninety-degree angles. Rest your arms on the floor outstretched at forty-five-degree angles, with your palms up. Let your back settle into the floor, and breathe from your diaphragm (that is, do stomach breathing). Keep your abs relaxed (an easy test is to see if your stomach is rising and falling with each breath).

OWN IT: Hold this position for five minutes.

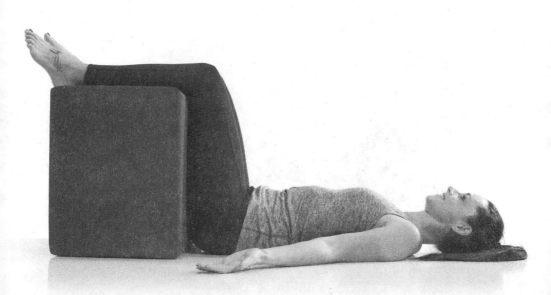

Frog

KNOW IT: Releases the powerful thigh and groin muscles to allow the pelvis to settle into a neutral position.

DO IT: Lie on your back with your feet pulled toward your torso and put the soles of your feet together, letting your knees turn out. Make sure your feet are centered in the middle of your body. Press your big toes and heels together to hold gentle pressure throughout the exercise. Your lower back doesn't have to be flat on the floor, but you should not feel pain in your back. Don't press on your knees. Just relax so you can feel a comfortable stretch in your inner thighs and groin.

OWN IT: Hold for two minutes.

Foot Circles and Point Flexes

KNOW IT: Increases ankle mobility and restores balance to the muscles of the lower extremity.

DO IT: Lie on your back with one leg extended flat on the floor and the other bent toward your chest. Your hip and knee should be at a ninety-degree angle. Clasp your hands behind your bent knee while you circle your foot clockwise twenty times (your other foot should be on the floor with your toes pointed to the ceiling; don't let the toes of the straight leg point off to either side). Reverse the direction of the circling foot and repeat twenty times. Change feet and repeat. Keep your knee still throughout the movement. For Point Flexes, stay in the same position on your back with one leg extended and the other bent. Bring your toes back toward the shin. Then, reverse direction to point the foot.

OWN IT: Do twenty flexes on each side.

Calf/Hamstring Stretch

KNOW IT: Restores balance to all the muscles from the hip to the foot.

DO IT: For the Calf Stretch, lie on your back with your knees bent and feet on the floor about hip-width apart. Use a belt or a strap with a loop to encircle the ball of your foot. Tighten your thigh while pulling your toes back with the strap; keep your leg straight and hoist it to about a forty-five-degree angle. Keep your shoulders relaxed.

OWN IT: Hold for thirty seconds on each side.

DO IT: For the Hamstring Stretch, use the same position but place the loop around the arch of the foot. Pull your entire leg toward your body, keeping it straight and your thigh muscle tight. Don't let your butt lift off the floor.

OWN IT: Hold for thirty seconds, and repeat on the other side.

Static Extension

KNOW IT: Improves pelvic and spine imbalance to improve load joint function.

DO IT: Kneel on a block or ottoman with your hands on the floor. Shift your hips forward six to eight inches so that your hips are slightly in front of your knees. Work your hands out in front of you until your hands are directly under your shoulders. Let your back and head drop toward the floor and your shoulder blades come together. Relax your abs. Try to tilt your butt toward the ceiling and notice the pronounced arch in your lower back.

OWN IT: Hold for one or two minutes.

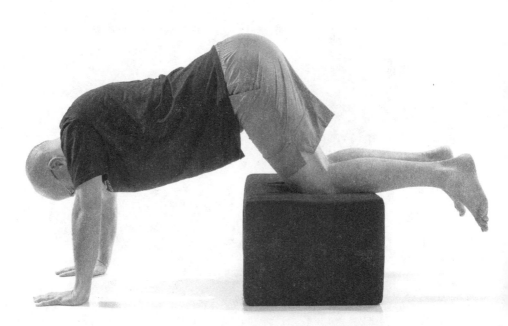

Air Bench

KNOW IT: Puts the hips, knees, and ankles simultaneously into flexion while they are under load.

DO IT: Stand with your back to a wall, and press your hips and the small of your back into the wall while walking your feet forward and sliding into a sitting position. Stop just before your hips reach a ninety-degree angle. Your knees should also be close to a ninety-degree angle, but your ankles should be just slightly forward of your knees. **Note:** If you feel pain in your knees, raise your body up the wall to relieve the pressure. Make sure your lower back is pressed against the wall and keep it pressed against the wall throughout the exercise. You should feel your quadriceps working along the top of the thigh.

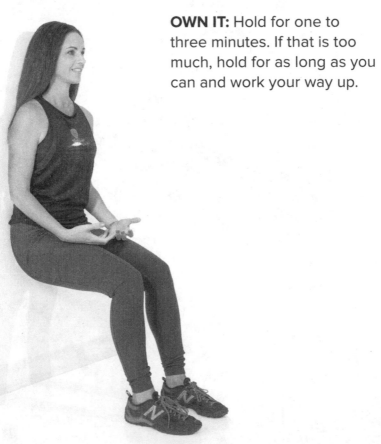

OWN IT: Hold for one to three minutes. If that is too much, hold for as long as you can and work your way up.

The Menu for Ankles

Standing Arm Circles...................... 80

Sitting Heel Raises with Block......... 82

Abduction-Adduction with
Narrow and Wide Feet.................. 83

Static Wall..................................... 84

Cats and Dogs............................... 85

Static Extension............................. 86

Cross-Crawling.............................. 87

Foot Circles and Point Flexes 88

Standing Arm Circles

KNOW IT: Strengthens the muscles of the upper back and shoulders, and balances the top of the kinetic chain and pelvis.

DO IT: Stand with your head up, feet squared, and arms at your sides. Put your hands in the golfer's grip (see opposite). Raise your arms out to the sides, keeping your elbows straight, palms down, and thumbs pointing forward. Lift your arms until they are level with your shoulders. If one shoulder wants to wobble forward or pop up, lower both until they stay level. Now squeeze your shoulder blades together slightly, and rotate your arms forward in a six-inch-diameter circle (you should be moving in the same direction as the thumbs are pointing). Then, reverse the circle by turning your palms up and thumbs back. Always make the circles in the direction that the thumb is pointing. Don't let your arms drop as you do the circles.

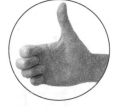

Use the "golfer's grip," see opposite page for details.

OWN IT: Do fifty with your palms down and fifty with your palms up.

Golfer's Grip

Your hands should be in golfer's grip, with your fingers curled, knuckles flexed, and thumbs extended. Your wrist, hand, and fingers up to the first knuckle should be in a straight line. The top of your fingers should be bent, and you should try to "squeeze" your palm with your fingertips, but don't allow your first knuckle to move out of alignment with your hand and wrist.

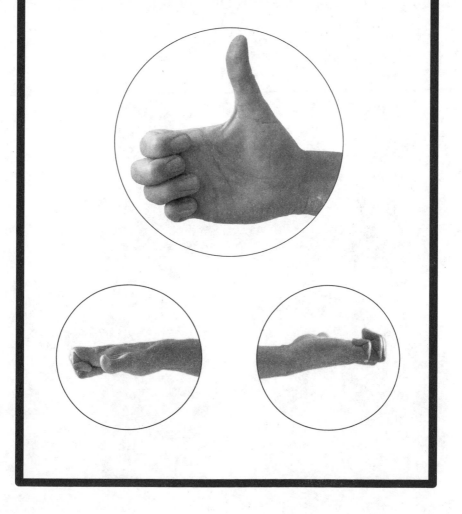

Sitting Heel Raises with Block

KNOW IT: Helps to coordinate movement of the entire lower extremity.

DO IT: Sit on the edge of a chair or bench, and arch your lower back by rolling your hips forward. Place a pillow or foam block between your knees and gently squeeze the block. Your toes should remain pointed straight ahead and your big toe should remain the center point of contact with the floor throughout the motion. Raise your heels. Don't push off your toes; instead, use your hip flexor muscles (imagine your toes are resting on eggshells to keep them relaxed).

OWN IT: Do three sets of ten repetitions.

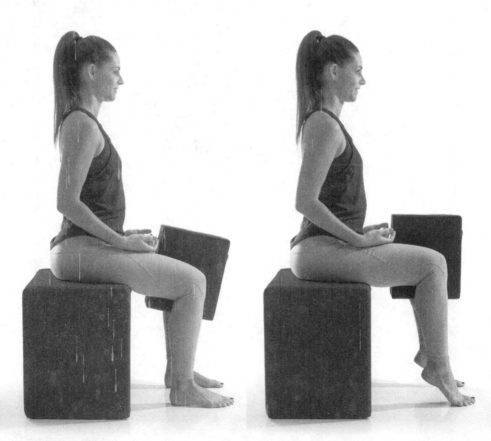

Abduction-Adduction with Narrow and Wide Feet

KNOW IT: Helps promote femur rotation and reduces imbalance in the pelvis and torso.

DO IT: Lie on your back with your knees bent at a ninety-degree angle and your feet flat on a wall. Keep your feet parallel, spaced about three inches apart, and pointed to the ceiling. Keep your upper body relaxed, with your palms up and your arms flat on the floor at about a forty-five-degree angle from your body. Bring your knees together slowly until they touch. Keep your feet pointed straight at the ceiling.

Bring your knees apart slowly so that your feet roll out to the sides. The bottoms of your feet will come off of the wall, but the outsides of your feet should remain touching the wall. Return your knees to the start position. Repeat the movement, but with your feet about twenty-four inches apart, bringing your knees together and then apart. Make sure your knees are meeting at the center line of your body when you bring them together.

OWN IT: Do two sets of ten repetitions of each position.

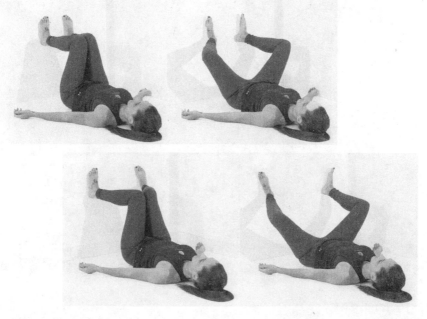

Static Wall

KNOW IT: Engages and balances the muscles in the front of the thighs, lower legs, and pelvis.

DO IT: Lie on your back and place your legs straight up against a wall hip-width apart. Get your butt and hamstrings as close to the wall as you can (the smaller the gap, the better), keeping your legs straight. If your knees are bent, slide back until you can keep them straight. Tighten your thighs and flex your feet, pulling your toes down toward the floor. Keep these muscles engaged throughout the exercise.

OWN IT: Hold for three to five minutes.

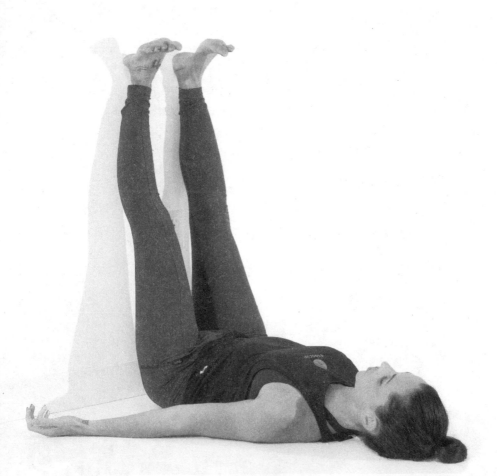

Cats and Dogs

KNOW IT: Works the hips, spine, shoulders, and neck in coordinated flexion-extension.

DO IT: Get down on the floor on your hands and knees. Make sure your knees are aligned with your hips, and your wrists with your shoulders. Your legs should be parallel with each other, and your feet relaxed with your toes pointed. Make sure your weight is distributed evenly. Smoothly round your back upward as your head tucks under to create a curve that runs from your butt to your neck (this is the cat with the arched back). Smoothly sway back down while bringing your head up and arching the back in the opposite direction (this is the gimme-a-treat dog). Try to initiate the movement with your pelvis. Make the two moves flow continuously back and forth rather than keeping them distinct and choppy.

OWN IT: Do one set of ten.

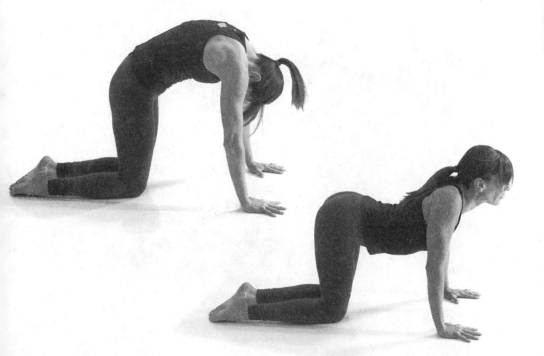

Static Extension

KNOW IT: Improves pelvic and spine imbalance to improve load joint function.

DO IT: Kneel on a block or ottoman with your hands on the floor. Shift your hips forward six to eight inches so that your hips are slightly in front of your knees. Work your hands out in front of you until your hands are directly under your shoulders. Let your back and head drop toward the floor and your shoulder blades come together. Relax your abs. Try to tilt your butt toward the ceiling and notice the pronounced arch in your lower back.

OWN IT: Hold for one or two minutes.

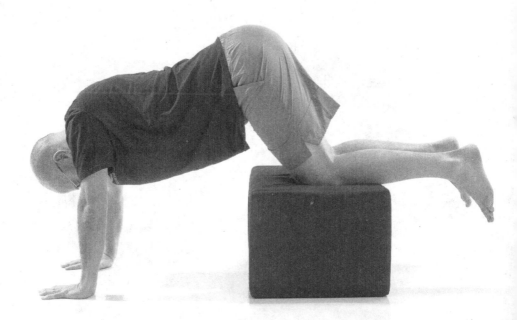

Cross-Crawling

KNOW IT: Promotes proper and coordinated flexion and extension of the hips and shoulders simultaneously.

DO IT: Lie on your back with both of your legs stretched out, feet flexed, and your arms resting beside your body (palms down). Simultaneously, raise one arm and the opposite leg. Your arm remains locked straight as you take it overhead until it reaches the floor (now extended straight above your head with your palm facing the ceiling). At the same time you are moving your arm, bend the opposite leg, bringing the knee up toward the chest until the hip is at a right angle. Your knee should also be at a ninety-degree angle to finish the movement. Simultaneously, return your arm and bent leg to the starting position and switch sides.

OWN IT: Do two sets of ten repetitions on each side.

Foot Circles and Point Flexes

KNOW IT: Increases ankle mobility and restores balance to the muscles of the lower extremity.

DO IT: Lie on your back with one leg extended flat on the floor and the other bent toward your chest. Your hip and knee should be at a ninety-degree angle. Clasp your hands behind your bent knee while you circle your foot clockwise twenty times (your other foot should be on the floor with your toes pointed to the ceiling; don't let the toes of the straight leg point off to either side). Reverse the direction of the circling foot and repeat twenty times. Change feet and repeat. Keep your knee still throughout the movement. For Point Flexes, stay in the same position on your back with one leg extended and the other bent. Bring your toes back toward the shin. Then, reverse direction to point the foot.

OWN IT: Do twenty flexes on each side.

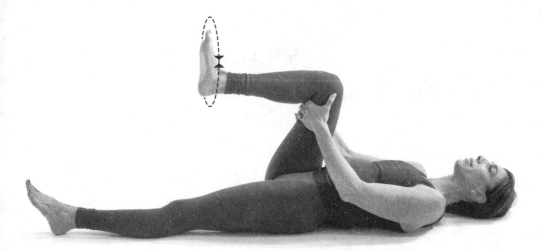

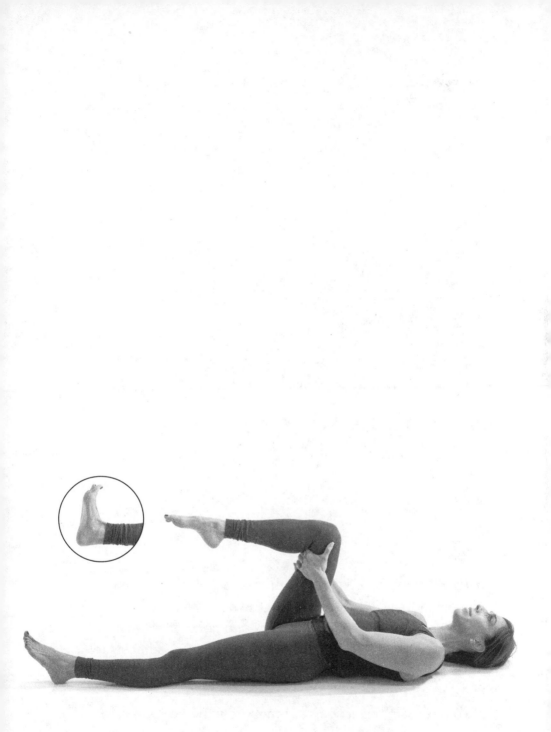

7

Knees: The Biology of Benders

Simply put, the knee provides a very elegant solution to a diabolically difficult problem. The muscles around the hip are critically important when it comes to generating the force needed to power movement. The ankle (via the foot) acts to transfer that force into the ground. The hip and the ankle move at vastly different speeds. Their gears, if you will, vary in size. Their muscular power sources range from the equivalent of jet engines to rubber bands. Hooking them together is at once madness and pure genius, making the knee among the best transmissions ever made.

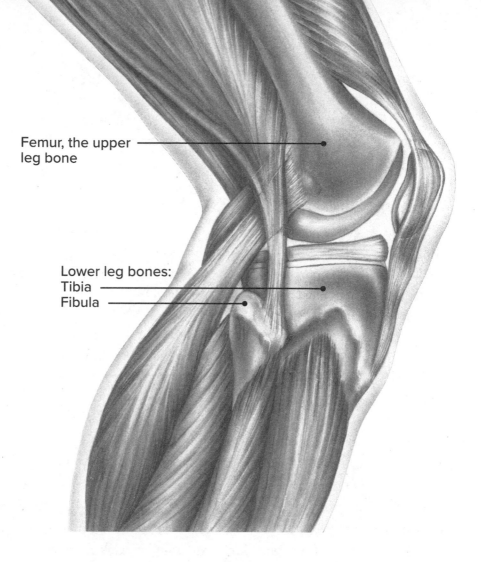

Femur, the upper
leg bone

Lower leg bones:
Tibia
Fibula

The knee is the junction of the upper leg bone (the femur) and the lower leg bones (the tibia and the fibula). The knee joint is primarily designed to move in one plane—hinging from front to back. But all joints are built with some degree of rotation and lateral movement. In this respect, joints resemble a gimbal, a device that keeps a ship's compass level as the vessel pitches and rolls with the waves. Of course, unlike a gimbal, the range of motion of our joints is restricted by surrounding muscles, ligaments, and joint capsules. After all, something must prevent us from collapsing into a heap of bones and muscles whenever we bend over to tie our shoes.

When it comes to flexion and extension, our knee has an impressive range of motion. But when it comes to twisting and side-to-side movement, the knee is more limited. Our knee allows for a small amount of rotation when flexed. Limited wiggle room for unexpected side-to-side motions helps to protect the supporting ligaments from injury, but once locked in extension, our knee is not designed to rotate. This single-plane mobility makes the knee inherently very stable. This is optimal because while helping to move and support almost our entire body weight, the knee must also provide a stable connection between the hip and ankle.

Because our knee is designed to primarily flex and extend, there are limited muscles surrounding the joint to power lateral and twisting movements. Without that muscular backup, the knee ligaments stand alone as a last line of joint defense. There are few nearby muscles to recruit to resist unexpected lateral and rotational force. Ligaments have a lot of strength but they do not have the elasticity to accommodate for large amounts of unexpected movement. Too much rotation or lateral force at the knee falls directly to the ligaments, and unlike muscles, ligaments cannot stretch very much before they tear. That is why knee injuries are so frequently associated with season-ending devastation.

If you have ever watched a karate black belt break a piece of wood in half, you can likely visualize why knee injuries can be such a calamity. Almost invariably, if the karate ninja is successful, the board breaks in the center. Why? Because the force required to break the board is reduced the farther you move from its supported ends. If you think of the leg as a board, the knee is at the center, located the farthest from the leg's supported anchors—the foot being anchored to the ground and the hip being anchored to the torso. The knee is not weak, but if you play the odds, physics tells you the knee is simply more vulnerable than the hip or ankle.

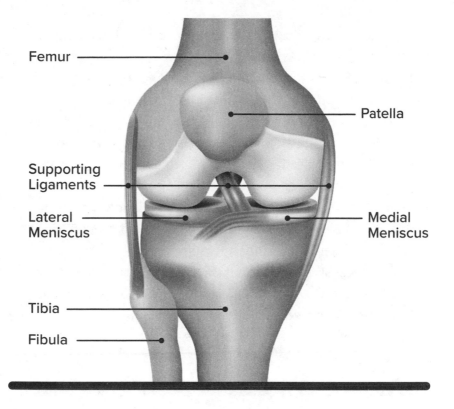

Femur

Patella

Supporting Ligaments

Lateral Meniscus

Medial Meniscus

Tibia

Fibula

Mirror Image Gone Awry

Except for the spine and the skull, the human musculoskeletal system has two of everything. The two halves of the body, to the left and the right of the spine, are functionally identical. Both sides are designed to operate in the same manner. When they don't, the balance and health of the entire musculoskeletal system are affected. The knee is no exception. Absent a nasty football tackle or downhill skiing crash, most knee pain is the result of imbalance. When was the last time someone told you that both their knees hurt in the exact same way, at the exact same spot, after the exact same activity? Think about that— really—I'll wait . . .

The answer, if we are honest, is never. The reason is simple.

Imbalance creates most knee problems, and when it comes to the human musculoskeletal system, imbalance is, by its very nature, asymmetrical. Even the pain that lingers after sudden traumatic injuries is often produced by imbalance. After broken bones and torn ligaments have healed, many people with traumatic knee injuries continue to experience pain. Often, lingering imbalances that existed before the injury, or weaknesses that developed during the healing process, stand in the way of becoming pain free. Correcting imbalance is essential to long-lasting pain relief, but it is also essential to preventing new problems and injuries further down the road.

The impressive thing about the body's design is that it is built to tolerate violations of its standard operating procedure. The most common deviation involves substituting other muscles involved in rotation and side-to-side movements

What's with the Kneecap?

Located along the front of the knee joint, the patella (aka the kneecap) rests along the front part of the knee. We can walk without a patella, so what is the point of having one at all? The answer is yet another testament to the body's innately brilliant design. This triangular bone sits in the middle of a long tendon connecting the quadriceps muscle to the lower leg. Acting like the fulcrum of a lever, the patella moves this tendon farther away from the knee joint and increases the strength of our quadriceps by 30 to 50 percent. That allows us to extend the knee with less effort, making movement more efficient.

to compensate for weakness in the muscles responsible for moving us from front to back. This works all right for a limited time at joints with more multidirectional leeway, but the knee is designed to be largely unidirectional. The knee's stability largely depends upon being free of rotational movement when straight.

Since the musculoskeletal system behaves as a unit, compensation with excessive rotation and lateral movement anywhere in the lower extremity must be transmitted through the knee, and that is a recipe for disaster. It is not a coincidence that the knee is the most commonly replaced joint. Our sedentary lifestyle commonly causes weakness in the muscles designed to power forward and backward movements. Such weakness makes us increasingly dependent on rotation and lateral movements to get around, and the knee has the least amount of built-in tolerance for this type of excessive movement.

Letting Go of Accidents Happen

Healthy knees need one thing: alignment with the other load joints. Knees rarely have problems if they are aligned and allowed to work with the hips and ankles. But we have persuaded ourselves that knees are accidents waiting to happen, time bombs ready to explode at any moment. True accidents and unpredictable explosions do occur, but thankfully they are more the exception than the rule. More often, what we construe as misfortunes, mishaps, and misadventures are really secondary consequences of misalignment, dysfunction, and imbalance. If we are convinced that pain is the result of an isolated accident and a vulnerable joint, we will mistakenly believe just fixing the damage is enough. The underlying dysfunction and misalignment will remain, unaddressed and primed to cause future accidents and misfortunes down the road.

See for Yourself

Aside from pain, the two most recognizable signs of knee problems appear in the feet and the kneecaps. Don't take my word for it—see for yourself!

Stand in front of a full-length mirror wearing a pair of shorts and no shoes. Don't try to straighten up—stand naturally. Start by looking at your feet. Functional feet should point directly at the mirror. Odds are one or both of your feet point off to the side (either out like a duck, or in like a pigeon). Now look at your knees. Functional knees are lined up directly underneath the

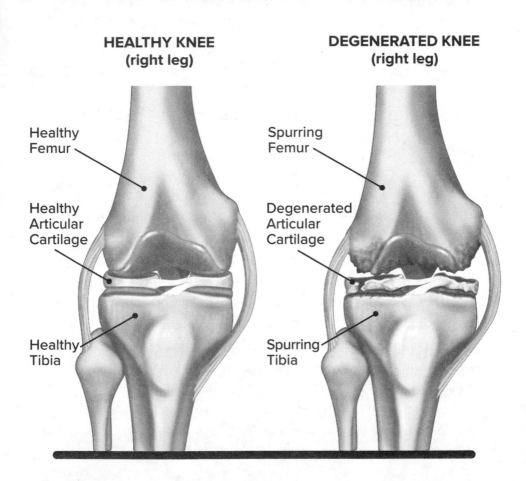

HEALTHY KNEE
(right leg)

Healthy Femur

Healthy Articular Cartilage

Healthy Tibia

DEGENERATED KNEE
(right leg)

Spurring Femur

Degenerated Articular Cartilage

Spurring Tibia

hips and directly above the ankles. Imagine a straight line connecting the joints. Better yet—take a marking pen and place a dot at the center of each kneecap and another front and center on the ankle. If you have a dysfunction, the dot on the kneecap will rest either on the inside or the outside of the invisible line that should run vertically between the two dots. If you back up and walk toward the mirror, you will probably see the dots gyrate wildly, moving inside and outside that invisible vertical line. Any (and all) deviations from that invisible vertical line represent imbalance within the musculoskeletal system.

Understanding Arthritis

Given its largely unidirectional design, the knee is incredibly efficient at absorbing symmetrical force. The cartilage, a smooth protective coat that sits on top of the bones within the joint, is designed to buffer impact and the friction generated as the joint moves. Dysfunction creates asymmetrical force across the joint. The cartilage can withstand symmetrical force indefinitely, but asymmetrical force is the equivalent of cartilage kryptonite. As the cartilage breaks down, the underlying surfaces of the femur and tibia become exposed. The smooth glide of cartilage is replaced by the harsh grind of exposed bone. Arthritis and pain ensue.

The body responds to pain and adapts, shifting force to an unworn area of the joint cartilage. But that change exposes a new area of the joint to asymmetrical force, and the cycle begins anew. Joint replacements can eliminate the worn bony surfaces, but they do nothing to fix the underlying dysfunction and asymmetrical force distribution. There is lots of ongoing research about whether cartilage can regenerate, but there is little debate that restoring symmetrical force distribution and eliminating dysfunction can help reduce pain and prevent further joint damage.

Menisci-Mysteries

Meniscus injuries are common—too common, really. And many of those injuries are entirely preventable. The meniscus is a wedge of cartilage that helps to stabilize the knee. The top of the tibia has two flat plateaus where either side of the femur can rest. The bottom of the femur is round, meaning only a small portion of the femur can actually be in contact with the flat tibia at any given time. The meniscus fills the space left around the bony surfaces of the joint, increasing the area of contact between the upper leg and the lower leg. This aids with weight distribution and force absorption and helps guide and stabilize knee movement.

Rotation and side-to-side movement in the upper or lower leg changes how the femur sits on the tibia. With the femur no longer centered over the tibial plateaus, the extra burden of stabilizing the joint falls to the meniscus and surrounding ligaments. This stress reduces the amount of additional unexpected movement the meniscus can withstand before tearing.

Most people who tear their meniscus have some abnormal rotation or side-to-side movement in their leg. Correcting that imbalance reduces the risk of meniscus injury. And after a meniscus injury, correcting imbalance reduces pain and alleviates unnecessary additional stress on the injured area, giving the body the opportunity to heal.

Joint Effusions

Joint effusion is just the medical term for joint swelling. Each of our joints is contained within a capsule. That capsule houses synovial fluid, a friction-reducing substance that bathes all of our joints and helps facilitate smooth motion. When the knee (or any joint) is injured, the joint often swells. The additional fluid in the joint capsule acts like a protective airbag, helping to

The Meniscus

The meniscus is a wedge of cartilage that sits on both sides of the knee. This critical piece of tissue helps to absorb force, distribute load, and stabilize the knee. The meniscus is shaped like a chock block, filling the space between the femur and the tibia to limit excess movement within the joint. Without the meniscus, the muscles around the knee would have to do more work to keep the round femur from sliding off the flat tibia.

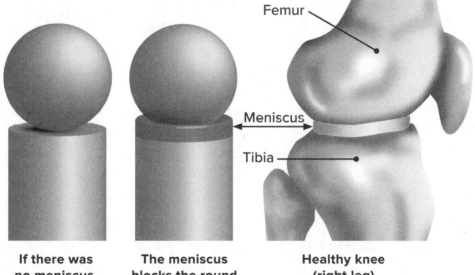

Femur

Meniscus

Tibia

If there was no meniscus, the round femur could freely slide off the flat tibia.

The meniscus blocks the round femur from freely sliding off the tibia.

Healthy knee (right leg)

The meniscus also increases the amount of contact between the upper leg and the lower leg, which aids in force distribution. Without the meniscus, only a small portion of the round femur would be in contact with the flat tibia. The meniscus allows for the forces generated during movement to be distributed over a larger surface area, reducing the amount of wear and tear any one particular spot must withstand.

buffer and restrict the movement within the joint. But the joint capsule is not designed to stretch, and too much fluid within the joint results in pain.

When the cartilage of our joints is subject to asymmetrical stress, pieces of that cartilage can break off and begin floating around in our joint. This can be really problematic. That loose cartilage can further interfere with the finely calibrated movement of the joint, like gravel thrown into the cylinders of an engine as the pistons are pumping up and down. Just like an engine, the joint can end up frozen in place. The cartilage can become caught between the moving bones, locking the joint and preventing further movement. Unfortunately, whereas engine pistons have no nerve endings, our bones have plenty, and jamming a piece of cartilage firmly between two bones hurts—a lot.

A Word About Knee Braces

Joint braces of any kind do one thing—restrict movement. There are instances where that restriction is necessary to allow the body time to heal, such as following a broken bone or an ACL reconstruction surgery. Outside of those circumstances, restricting joint movement generally does more damage in the long run by making the muscles and joints less capable of moving properly. A knee brace changes the interactions of the femur, tibia, and fibula, the bones that make up the joint. Restricted femur movement at the knee limits femur movement at the hip, instantly changing the dynamics of the hip, pelvis, back, and shoulder. One restrictive change has a ripple effect on movement patterns throughout the body, and aches and pains generally follow close behind. Seriously, if you ever need to demonstrate the snowball effect, just lock your knee in a brace and walk around, taking note of all the little niggles that start to emerge.

The Menu for Knees

(If One or Both of Your Femurs Are Externally Rotated)

Flexion Knee Pillow Squeezes.......103

Static Back....................................104

Cats and Dogs..............................105

Static Extension............................106

Standing Quad Stretch..................107

Standing Forward Bend.................108

Cats and Dogs..............................109

Progressive Supine Groin.............110

Flexion Knee Pillow Squeezes

KNOW IT: Helps the adductor muscles do their primary assignment, rather than trying to operate as gait muscles.

DO IT: Sit on the edge of a chair or bench. Pull your shoulders back, and make sure your knees and feet are in alignment with your hips. Relax your stomach muscles (let them hang). Place a pillow between your knees. Using your inner thighs, squeeze the pillow and release it gently. Your feet should stay parallel to each other, and your knees should stay in line with your hips even as you squeeze (you may need to fold the pillow to give it thickness). Don't let your stomach or upper back engage in the movement.

OWN IT: Do three sets of ten repetitions.

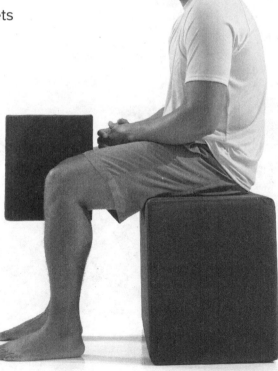

Static Back

KNOW IT: Settles your hips and back, releasing the compensating muscles that interfere with balance and functional movement.

DO IT: Lie on your back with both legs bent at right angles on a chair or block. Your hips should also be at ninety-degree angles. Rest your arms on the floor outstretched at forty-five-degree angles, with your palms up. Let your back settle into the floor, and breathe from your diaphragm (that is, do stomach breathing). Keep your abs relaxed (an easy test is to see if your stomach is rising and falling with each breath).

OWN IT: Hold this position for five minutes.

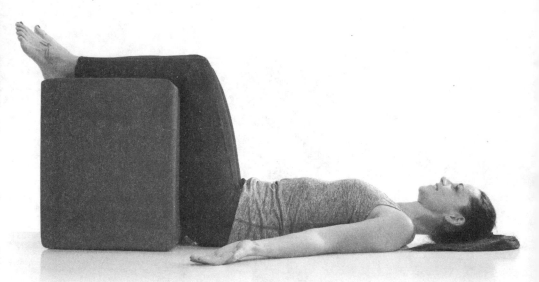

Cats and Dogs

KNOW IT: Works the hips, spine, shoulders, and neck in coordinated flexion-extension.

DO IT: Get down on the floor on your hands and knees. Make sure your knees are aligned with your hips, and your wrists with your shoulders. Your legs should be parallel with each other, and your feet relaxed with your toes pointed. Make sure your weight is distributed evenly. Smoothly round your back upward as your head tucks under to create a curve that runs from your butt to your neck (this is the cat with the arched back). Smoothly sway back down while bringing your head up and arching the back in the opposite direction (this is the gimme-a-treat dog). Try to initiate the movement with your pelvis. Make the two moves flow continuously back and forth rather than keeping them distinct and choppy.

OWN IT: Do one set of ten.

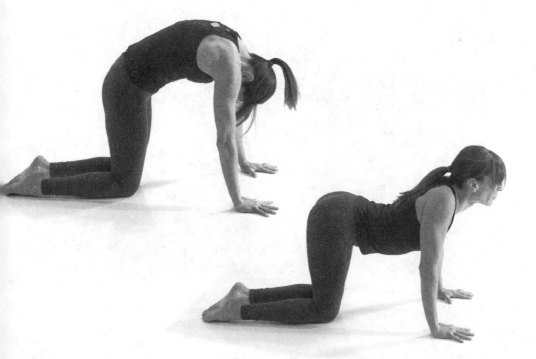

Static Extension

KNOW IT: Improves pelvic and spine imbalance to improve load joint function.

DO IT: Kneel on a block or ottoman with your hands on the floor. Shift your hips forward six to eight inches so that your hips are slightly in front of your knees. Work your hands out in front of you until your hands are directly under your shoulders. Let your back and head drop toward the floor and your shoulder blades come together. Relax your abs. Try to tilt your butt toward the ceiling and notice the pronounced arch in your lower back.

OWN IT: Hold for one or two minutes.

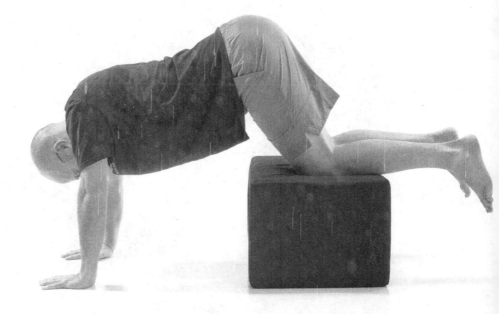

Standing Quad Stretch

KNOW IT: Helps to balance the quadriceps and hamstring muscles to balance pelvis and torso position.

DO IT: Stand on one foot and bend the other leg back, placing the top of the foot on a block or the back of a chair. Let the ankle relax so the foot is pointed. The height will dictate the amount of stretch in the quadriceps. Keep your hips and shoulders square. Tighten the thigh muscle on the straight leg and try to keep your bent knee directly underneath your hip. Tuck your hips under to feel the stretch. If necessary, hold on to something for balance.

OWN IT: Hold for one minute on each side.

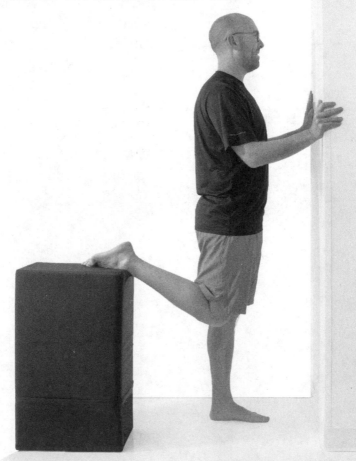

Standing Forward Bend

KNOW IT: Allows for coordinated movement on both sides of the trunk and pelvis and balances the muscles along the front and back of the body, stabilizing the pelvis.

DO IT: Stand with your feet pointing straight ahead and place your palms on your lower back/upper butt area. Tilt your pelvis forward to place an exaggerated arch in your lower back while pulling your elbows and shoulder blades together behind you. Keeping the elbows back, begin bending forward from the hips. Keep the hips in line with the knees and ankles (don't stick your butt out behind your legs). Keep the lower back arched as you bend over from the hips, stopping where you can maintain the arch. Tighten your thighs to lock your knees straight, and move your body weight to the balls of your feet.

OWN IT: Hold this position for one minute.

Cats and Dogs

KNOW IT: Works the hips, spine, shoulders, and neck in coordinated flexion-extension.

DO IT: Get down on the floor on your hands and knees. Make sure your knees are aligned with your hips, and your wrists with your shoulders. Your legs should be parallel with each other, and your feet relaxed with your toes pointed. Make sure your weight is distributed evenly. Smoothly round your back upward as your head tucks under to create a curve that runs from your butt to your neck (this is the cat with the arched back). Smoothly sway back down while bringing your head up and arching the back in the opposite direction (this is the gimme-a-treat dog). Try to initiate the movement with your pelvis. Make the two moves flow continuously back and forth rather than keeping them distinct and choppy.

OWN IT: Do one set of ten.

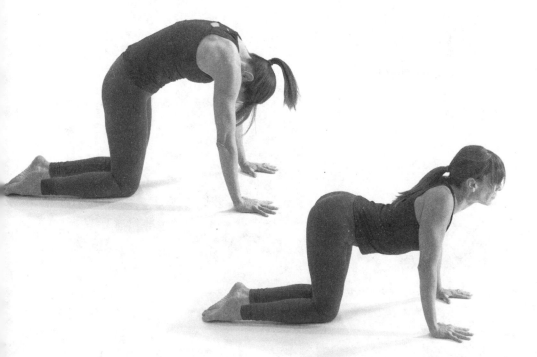

Progressive Supine Groin

KNOW IT: Allows for proper flexion and extension of the leg while reducing compensating side-to-side and rotational motions.

DO IT: Lie on your back with one leg resting on a block or chair, your knee bent at a ninety-degree angle, while the other leg is extended on a small stepladder, a stack of books, or something of a similar height (so that your back and hips are flat on the floor). Prop the outside of your foot on the extended leg to prevent it from rolling out. Let the leg rest at this top level for three to five minutes. Ideally, your lower back should come to rest flat against the floor before moving on. Lower your extended foot about five to eight inches and repeat for three to five minutes. Continue to progressively lower your extended foot five to eight inches at a time until your foot is resting against the floor. Again, let the leg rest along the floor until your lower back rests flat on the floor. Don't try to flatten your back. Let it happen naturally.

OWN IT: Hold each position for three minutes, and repeat on the opposite side.

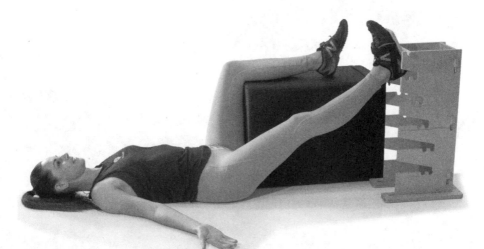

These images depict Progressive Supine Groin using the Egoscue tower, a tool specifically designed for the exercise. You can complete the exercise without the tower, as described above.

The Menu for Knees

(If One or Both of Your Femurs Are Internally Rotated)

Standing Wall with Block...............113

Wall Stork 114

Cats and Dogs................................115

Lying Supine...................................116

Modified Floor Block 117

Cats and Dogs................................118

Air Bench..119

Standing Wall with Block

KNOW IT: Promotes proper positioning of all load joints.

DO IT: Stand at a wall with your heels, hips, and upper back against the wall. Place a small block or pillow between your knees. Apply gentle pressure, just enough to hold the pillow in place; do not push into it. It's okay if your head is not against the wall. Stand in a relaxed position and let your head rest naturally. With enough time, your head will move back on its own; don't force it. Relax your stomach and your arms and allow your body to adjust to this new position. Keep your thighs tight so that your knees are locked in a straight, or extended, position. Remember to keep your feet pointed straight ahead and your stomach relaxed throughout.

OWN IT: Hold for six to eight minutes.

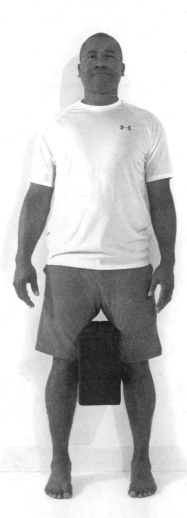

Wall Stork

KNOW IT: Strengthens independent movement of the hips and balances the pelvis, torso, and lower extremity.

DO IT: Stand with your back against the wall with your feet hip-width apart, pointing straight ahead. Your heels, hips, and upper back should be against the wall. Place one foot on a chair in front of you. Your knee should be bent to ninety degrees, thigh parallel to floor. Make sure that your foot is pointed straight. Do not allow the standing leg to bend or shift to the side. (Your hip, knee, and ankle should stay in a straight line.) Tighten the thigh muscle of the straight leg. Keep the shoulder and hip on the bent-leg side flat against the wall.

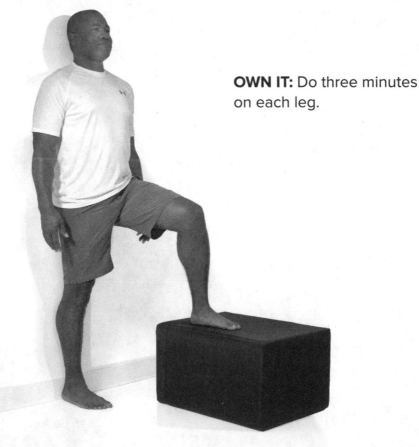

OWN IT: Do three minutes on each leg.

Cats and Dogs

KNOW IT: Works the hips, spine, shoulders, and neck in coordinated flexion-extension.

DO IT: Get down on the floor on your hands and knees. Make sure your knees are aligned with your hips, and your wrists with your shoulders. Your legs should be parallel with each other, and your feet relaxed with your toes pointed. Make sure your weight is distributed evenly. Smoothly round your back upward as your head tucks under to create a curve that runs from your butt to your neck (this is the cat with the arched back). Smoothly sway back down while bringing your head up and arching the back in the opposite direction (this is the gimme-a-treat dog). Try to initiate the movement with your pelvis. Make the two moves flow continuously back and forth rather than keeping them distinct and choppy.

OWN IT: Do one set of ten.

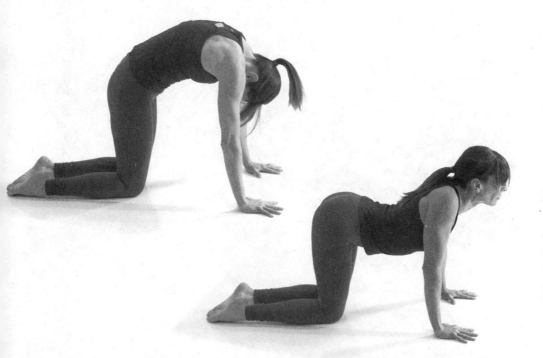

Lying Supine

KNOW IT: Helps to improve joint position and balance throughout the kinetic chain.

DO IT: Lie on your back with both legs straight and flat on the floor. Place a pillow or small block between your ankles/feet. Flex your toes back toward your hips, bending at the ankle joint. Keep gentle pressure along the block with the insides of your feet. Try to keep your upper body relaxed, with arms at a forty-five-degree angle to your body, palms up. Tighten the thigh muscles.

OWN IT: Hold for three to five minutes.

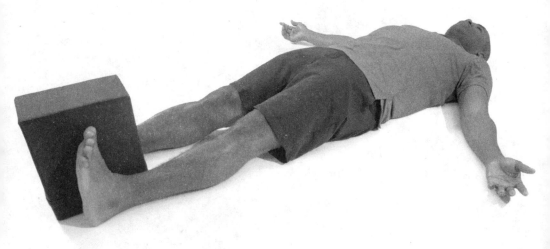

Modified Floor Block

KNOW IT: Coordinates shoulder, torso, and pelvic movement.

DO IT: Lie on your stomach with your forehead on the floor, your feet pigeon-toed (toes pointed, ankles relaxed), and your butt relaxed. Rest your forearms on six-inch-high blocks (lower if this causes discomfort) with your wrists relaxed and your hands dangling over the blocks' front edge. Your arms should extend at ninety degrees from the shoulder and should bend ninety degrees at the elbow. Make sure your shoulders are level from right to left. Breathe deeply and relax the upper body. Don't press your arms into the blocks. Let your stomach muscles relax.

OWN IT: Hold for six minutes.

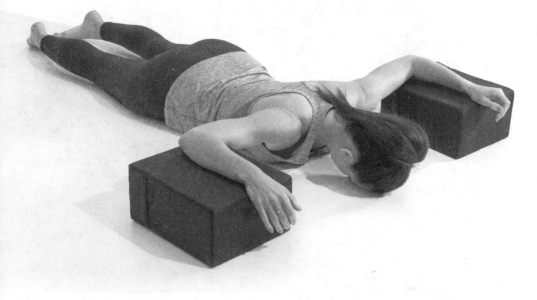

Cats and Dogs

KNOW IT: Works the hips, spine, shoulders, and neck in coordinated flexion-extension.

DO IT: Get down on the floor on your hands and knees. Make sure your knees are aligned with your hips, and your wrists with your shoulders. Your legs should be parallel with each other, and your feet relaxed with your toes pointed. Make sure your weight is distributed evenly. Smoothly round your back upward as your head tucks under to create a curve that runs from your butt to your neck (this is the cat with the arched back). Smoothly sway back down while bringing your head up and arching the back in the opposite direction (this is the gimme-a-treat dog). Try to initiate the movement with your pelvis. Make the two moves flow continuously back and forth rather than keeping them distinct and choppy.

OWN IT: Do one set of ten.

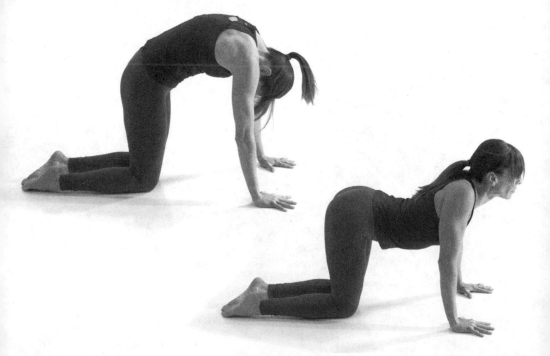

Air Bench

KNOW IT: Puts the hips, knees, and ankles simultaneously into flexion while they are under load.

DO IT: Stand with your back to a wall, and press your hips and the small of your back into the wall while walking your feet forward and sliding into a sitting position. Stop just before your hips reach a ninety-degree angle. Your knees should also be close to a ninety-degree angle, but your ankles should be just slightly forward of your knees. **Note:** If you feel pain in your knees, raise your body up the wall to relieve the pressure. Make sure your lower back is pressed against the wall and keep it pressed against the wall throughout the exercise. You should feel your quadriceps working along the top of the thigh.

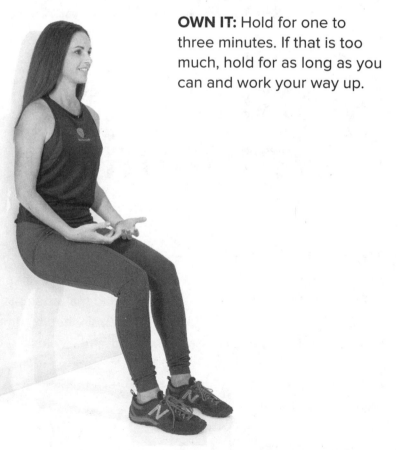

OWN IT: Hold for one to three minutes. If that is too much, hold for as long as you can and work your way up.

8

The Hip and the Pelvis:

Central Command

The pelvis is the MVP of musculoskeletal health and function. I don't make that statement lightly. After all, I firmly believe that the body functions as a unit and that attempts to isolate parts are largely a fool's errand. But when it comes to commanding the overall environment of the musculoskeletal system, the buck stops at the pelvis. And you don't need to take my word for it. The proof is you—visible instantly in your body's design.

The largest and strongest muscles in the body attach to the pelvis—the quadriceps, the hamstrings, the psoas, the glutes, the abdominal muscles, the back muscles. All our major movers link up with the pelvis. The pelvis is our biological equivalent of Grand Central Station. All movement passes through this critical junction. It is not too far-fetched to say that the pelvis is the body's other brain—that's how important it is. And judging by the amount of armored plating that nature has provided, the skull and the hip are definitely in the same league. Like the skull, our pelvis forms through the fusion of multiple bones. The result is a large, sturdy, protective structure built to endure incredible punishment while safeguarding essential functions.

United We Stand

Humans have the smallest base of support, the highest center of gravity, and the heaviest head of all mammals. We are inherently much less stable than our four-legged friends. Yet our upright position gives us many advantages, including a higher line of sight, a wider field of vision, and the freedom to use our arms and hands to perform other tasks. The pelvis is the linchpin of that upright posture. The pelvis is a no-frills, no-fuss bony basin that has a minimum of moving parts and a maximum of strength and stability. Without the pelvis as a platform and a fulcrum, our spine would be horizontal and we would move about on four legs instead of two.

Like any platform, the pelvis offers a stable surface that supports the spine and the upper body from below. As a fulcrum, the pelvis gives the spine leverage—an anchor from which it can be hoisted upright. The pelvis quite literally unites the musculoskeletal system, connecting the upper and lower halves of the body.

The pelvis connects with the lower body at the hip. The hip is a ball-and-socket joint, with the ball being the head of the femur (the large bone in the upper leg) and the socket being formed by the acetabulum. The acetabulum is a cup-like depression that sits on either side of the pelvis. The head of the femur fits tightly within the acetabulum. The hip is one of two ball-and-socket joints in the body, with the other being the shoulder. Ball-and-socket joints have more freedom of movement than any other joint type in the body. The hip allows the leg to swing from front to back and side to side, while simulta-

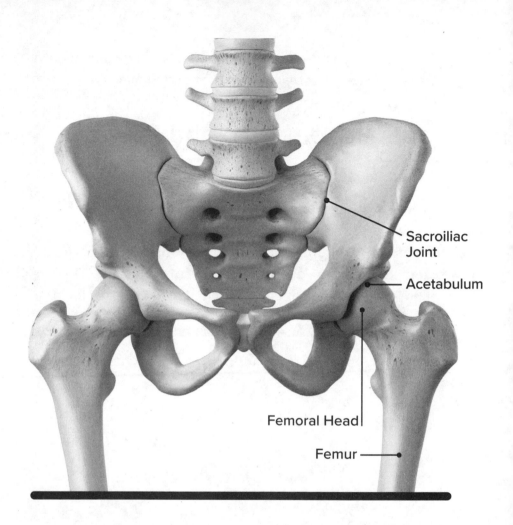

Sacroiliac Joint

Acetabulum

Femoral Head

Femur

neously allowing the leg to spin and rotate. This motion requires a large amount of surrounding musculature to both power movement and provide stability and support. Tough ligaments and powerful muscles hold the head of the femur in place and provide the stability necessary to bear the weight of the upper body while simultaneously powering the movement of the lower extremity.

Likewise, the pelvis connects with the upper body at the sacroiliac joints. These joints are located on the back of the pelvis and rest on either side of the spine. The sacroiliac joints have a small degree of mobility, but that motion is crucial to maintain balance and allow the independent movement of our lower extremities necessary for walking and running.

Understanding Hip and Pelvic Movement

Movement at our hip occurs by moving both the femur and the pelvis. Understanding how our femur moves is relatively straightforward. After all, we can literally watch it move. Lift your knee and bring your thigh up, toward your chest. That motion is what the femur does during hip flexion. Now lower

---

Understanding Pelvic Movement

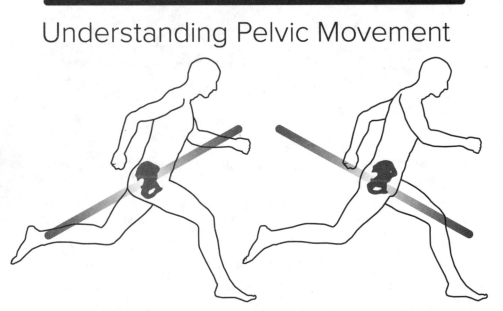

As we walk or run, we flex one hip while simultaneously extending the other. In doing so, one side of our pelvis tilts forward while the opposite side tilts backward. This seesaw-like movement allows us to independently move our lower extremities with less upper-body rotation and a longer stride length, making our two-legged ambulation much more efficient.

Mobile Unit

The shoulder tops the hip when it comes to the title of most mobile joint. Both are ball-and-socket joints. These joints anchor our arms and legs with our torso and allow for the immense mobility of our extremities. Unlike the upper extremity that remains largely unanchored during movement, the lower extremity is often anchored to the ground. The hip sacrifices some of its mobility in exchange for the stability necessary to support the weight of the body when standing and walking.

your thigh toward the floor and allow it to come behind your body, toward your back. This motion is what the femur does during hip extension.

The pelvis also moves during hip flexion and extension. Although it is less obvious, the mobility of the pelvis is critical to our ability to remain upright during movement. The easiest way to understand pelvic movement is to visualize two imaginary horizontal lines extending straight out from the hips, front to back: two parallel seesaws. The seesaws represent two walking or running hips. Let's say the left hip is in extension and the right hip is in flexion (the left leg is behind the body and the right leg is reaching for the ground in front of the body). The left seesaw is tipped forward and the right seesaw is tipped backward. As the right leg moves behind the body during the next stride, the right pelvis will tilt forward, with the left pelvis tipping backward as the left leg moves in front of the body. By alternating the tilt of the seesaws, the pelvis can maintain an overall neutral position, providing a flat surface to support and balance the spine and upper body even during movement.

A Musculoskeletal Silver Bullet

I am not a big believer in magic pills and silver bullets.
That said, restoring hip function is probably the closest thing
we've got when it comes to a miracle cure for musculoskeletal
problems. The numerous major muscles that connect
with the pelvis mean the hips play a central role in our mobility.
Hip misalignment has dramatic consequences from head to toe,
and eliminating hip dysfunction should be a top priority when
it comes to musculoskeletal health.

Our Modern Flexion Failure

Unfortunately, our modern motionless society fuels hip
dysfunction at such a feverish rate that we are blazing straight
for an inferno of pain. Sit, sit, and sit some more. Never before
in history have we spent so much time with our pelvis anchored
to a chair, driver's seat, or couch. Our hips are designed with
a lot of mobility, but that mobility requires balance, and balance
can be maintained only through movement. Cumulatively, we
spend so much time sitting, we all but live in a state of flexion.
The tug between flexion (bent) and extension (more upright)
becomes so lopsided that balance is practically an endangered
species.

When we sit, more often than not we conform to the chair.
That means that the arch of the lower back flattens, and then
reverses. As the top of the spine moves forward, the head and
shoulders move with it. The pelvis mirrors the changing curve
of the spine and tilts backward. The hips rest in flexion with the
femur running parallel to the ground along the seat of the chair.
When we spend enough time in this position, those major
muscles that drive our movement start to adapt. Some come
to rest in a position that is shorter than normal. Some come
to rest in a slightly stretched or lengthened state. Regardless,

Sit, Sit, and Sit Some More

Recent studies found the average American sits for 10 hours a day! Instead of our spine resembling an "S" (top), it starts to flatten out and mirror the shape of the chair. Our pelvis follows and begins to tilt posteriorly (bottom). To make matters even worse, we are sitting *so much* that our "C" shaped sedentary posture persists when we stand up and start moving.

sitting collapsed in a chair requires very minimal work, and our muscles become disengaged and weak. If flexion and extension were weights atop a pair of modern-posture scales, flexion would tip its scale straight to the ground.

As imbalance sets in, our hips and back slowly lose the strength and ability to move into extension. The body compensates with less efficient surrounding support muscles, using side-to-side and rotation movements as substitutes for extension. Our hips are pushed and pulled out of their proper positions, and movement of the lower body becomes compromised. Our pelvis comes to rest with a tilt rather than offering a neutral, flat surface upon which the spine can rest, and movement of the upper body becomes compromised. If I were to gamble on that musculoskeletal silver bullet, I would go all in on sitting less.

Beat Back Arthritis

The word *arthritis* spooks people, but it only means what it objectively denotes in Latin: inflammation of a joint. Hip arthritis, like that of the knee, results from asymmetrical force causing cartilage breakdown. Deteriorating cartilage tends to pit and crater. Through trial and painful error, the body quickly learns to navigate this lunar landscape with a minimum of suffering. Obeying the muscles, the ball and socket do their best to avoid the worst spots (the biggest craters) and limit contact with areas that cannot be avoided. Hip movement becomes dependent on an increasingly intricate, restricted, and demanding series of muscle improvisations. But here is the catch. Restricted movement places devastating point pressure on new areas of cartilage, leading to new pits and craters. Those new pits and craters further restrict movement and further concentrate pressure on what little cartilage remains. The only way to break this vicious cycle is to restore muscular balance and symmetrically distribute pressure across the joint surface.

The Body Is a Unit

Hip arthritis does not occur in a vacuum. The force placed upon the hip joint is influenced by all other joints in the body. Take hip replacements as an example. Almost 70 percent of

Hips Don't Lie

There is a well-publicized theory that potential male mates are more attracted to females with smaller waists and larger hips. From a strictly evolutionary standpoint, a male's interest in a female mate is strongly influenced by the odds of his own reproductive success. Numerous physical and physiological characteristics have been associated with this magical waist-hip ratio and scientists have theorized that males instinctively use this visual cue as a gauge of health and fertility.

Scientific theories on attractiveness aside, the position of the hips certainly plays a crucial role during childbirth. In order for a woman to naturally birth a child, the baby must pass through the woman's bony pelvis to make his or her grand entrance into the world. It is a tight fit, and the baby needs all the help he can get to successfully complete the journey. To help, the position of a woman's pelvis changes during pregnancy. The pelvis tilts forward and hormones increase the laxity of the supporting ligaments to expand the pelvic channel. Asymmetries in hip or pelvic position and limitations in hip and pelvic mobility can restrict the changes necessary to facilitate childbirth. A balanced, mobile pelvis is the best gift a mom can give her child to help set the baby up for a successful descent into the birth canal and a safer, easier birth.

people who undergo hip replacement surgery have that surgery done on their dominant side. Right-handed people are far more likely to have their right hip replaced than their left. Why? Upper-body imbalance affects shoulder position, which in turn affects hip position. We use our dominant hand far more often for repetitive tasks. Imbalance creates abnormal stress on the muscles, bones, and joints and that abnormal strain accumulates faster the more frequently we move in an unbalanced way.

It's Not Too Late

So, you have already had a hip replacement and completed your postoperative physical therapy. The E-cises recommended in this chapter are still very useful. Chances are, your hip went "bad" because of musculoskeletal dysfunctions that are still around. The muscles aren't replaced when an artificial hip is installed, and muscle pain is often responsible for much of the agony associated with a bad hip. Realigning your hips with the rest of your load joints will prevent unnecessary wear and tear on your new joint and prevent new symptoms from cropping up elsewhere.

The Menu for Hips/Pelvis

(No Pain, but with Motion Restriction)

Static Back with Knee
Pillow Squeezes 132

Hooklying Rocking Chair 133

Hip Lift 134

Pelvic Tilts 135

Foot Circles and Point Flexes 136

Floor Block 137

Active Wishbone 138

Kneeling Counter Stretch 139

Gravity Drop 140

Static Back with Knee Pillow Squeezes

KNOW IT: Helps to balance pelvis and torso to allow proper movement of the hip and proper rotation of the femur.

DO IT: Lie on your back with both legs bent at right angles on a chair or block. Your hips should also be at ninety-degree angles. Rest your arms on the floor outstretched at forty-five-degree angles, with your palms up. Let your back settle into the floor, and breathe from your diaphragm (that is, do stomach breathing). Keep your abs relaxed (an easy test is to see if your stomach is rising/falling with each breath). Hold for three minutes. Place a pillow between your knees. Using your inner thighs, squeeze the pillow and release, applying pressure evenly on either side of the block. Your feet should remain parallel to each other.

OWN IT: Hold static back for three minutes. Then do three sets of ten repetitions of knee pillow squeezes.

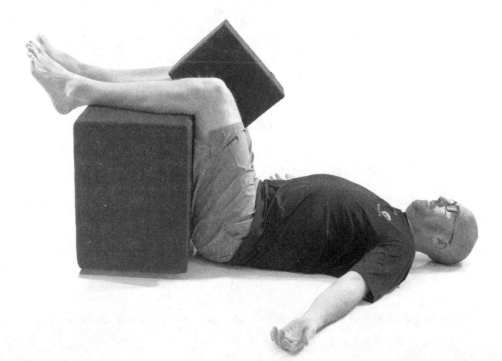

Hooklying Rocking Chair

KNOW IT: Improves range of motion in the ankle and coordinates the movement of the entire lower extremity.

DO IT: Lie on your back with your knees bent and your feet flat on the floor, pointed straight ahead. Your arms should be out to the sides at forty-five-degree angles, palms up. Place a pillow or block between your knees and keep light pressure against it. Keep your upper body relaxed. Roll both feet forward onto the ball of each foot (raising the heels off the ground). Keep your big toe engaged with the floor as you do so. Then roll both feet back onto the heel of each foot (raising the toes off the ground and pulling the foot back toward the shin). Keep gentle pressure against the block throughout the motion.

OWN IT: Do three sets of ten repetitions.

Hip Lift

KNOW IT: Helps to reduce pelvic disparity and to balance femur and torso position.

DO IT: Lie on your back with both knees bent and feet flat on the floor. Cross your right ankle over the left knee, allowing it to rest on your left thigh. Press your right knee out toward your opposite foot. While maintaining this position, lift your bent left leg toward your chest. Make sure your torso and shoulders stay evenly on the floor. Hold this position as you breathe. Check that your left knee, left hip, and left shoulder are all in the same plane. Continue to push the right knee away from your body. You should feel a stretch in the right hip.

OWN IT: Do one minute on each side.

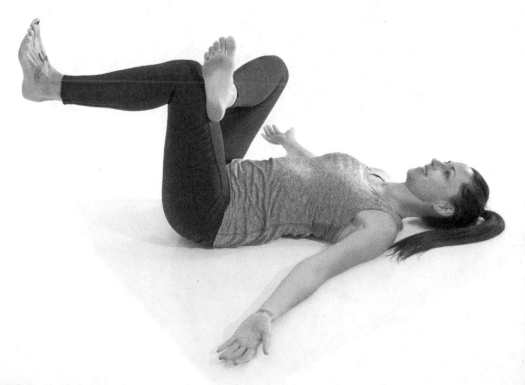

Pelvic Tilts

KNOW IT: Coordinates movement of the lower spine and pelvis.

DO IT: Lie on your back with your knees bent, feet flat on the floor, and arms out to the sides at ninety-degree angles. Roll your hips toward your torso to flatten your lower back into the floor. Do not lift your hips off the floor. Then roll your hips away to make your lower back arch off the floor, creating a space between the floor and your back. Do these rolls in a smooth and continuous motion, flattening your back into the floor and rolling the lower back off the floor by changing the tilt of your pelvis.

OWN IT: Do one set of ten repetitions.

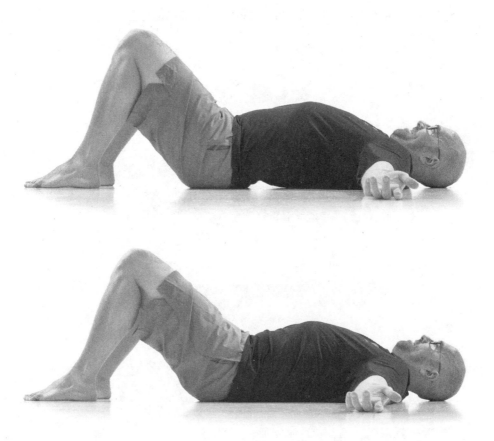

Foot Circles and Point Flexes

KNOW IT: Increases ankle mobility and restores balance to the muscles of the lower extremity.

DO IT: Lie on your back with one leg extended flat on the floor and the other bent toward your chest. Your hip and knee should be at a ninety-degree angle. Clasp your hands behind your bent knee while you circle your foot clockwise twenty times (your other foot should be on the floor with your toes pointed to the ceiling; don't let the toes of the straight leg point off to either side). Reverse the direction of the circling foot and repeat twenty times. Change feet and repeat. Keep your knee still throughout the movement. For Point Flexes, stay in the same position on your back with one leg extended and the other bent. Bring your toes back toward the shin. Then, reverse direction to point the foot.

OWN IT: Do twenty flexes on each side.

Floor Block

KNOW IT: Coordinates movement of the humerus and scapula and helps to balance the torso and spine.

DO IT: Lie on your stomach, facedown and arms over your head, with your elbows straight and feet pigeon-toed. Rest your forearms on six-inch blocks. Place your hands in a golfer's grip with your fingers curled, knuckles flexed, and thumbs extended, and point your thumbs toward the ceiling. Place your forehead on the floor and keep your neck, shoulder, butt, and stomach relaxed. Move your arms outward, away from your body, and continuously try to get more range throughout the exercise. Initiate the movement from your shoulders, not your elbows. Hold for one minute, then repeat with your arms at 10 o'clock and 2, and then again at 9 o'clock and 3.

Use the "golfer's grip," see page 81 for details.

OWN IT: Hold for one minute in each position.

Active Wishbone

KNOW IT: Reduces hip disparities and balances the pelvis and torso.

DO IT: Lie on your stomach with your forehead on your hands. Keep your palms on the floor with your fingers overlapping and elbows out to the sides. Keep your upper body relaxed. Bend your knees to bring your ankles toward your butt. Flex your feet by pulling your toes down toward the floor, and keep them flexed throughout. Squeeze your knees together. Keeping your feet flexed, slowly move your ankles out to the sides, rotating the femur and spreading the lower legs apart. Then bring the ankles back together. Keep your knees together throughout the movement. Slowly move your ankles/feet apart and then bring them back together using just the muscles of your hips.

OWN IT: Do three sets of ten repetitions.

Kneeling Counter Stretch

KNOW IT: Allows for symmetric spinal extension and balances the hips and shoulders from side to side.

DO IT: Kneel with your hips over your knees while extending your arms, palms down, on a chair or low table. Relax your torso so that the back seems as if it's trying to fall through your arms. Your hands should rest flat against the surface. Point your toes. Breathe deeply and try to continuously increase the curve in your lower back by tilting the pelvis forward.

OWN IT: Hold for one minute.

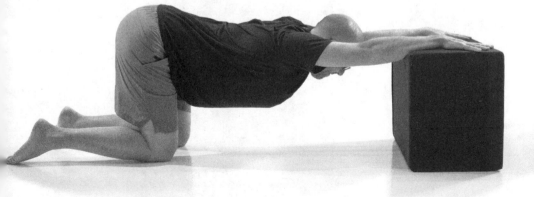

Gravity Drop

KNOW IT: Balances the rotation in the lower extremity and aligns the load joints.

DO IT: Wearing rubber-soled shoes for traction, stand on a step (facing upward) with your feet parallel and shoulder-width apart. With one hand, hold on to the railing for support, and edge backward until your heels are off the step and hanging in midair. Keep inching back so that more than half of the foot is off the step. Make sure your feet remain parallel, pointing straight ahead (and that they are hip-width apart). Let the weight of your body press down, lowering your heels. Keep your knees, hips, and shoulders in line with your ankles. Don't bend your knees. Tighten your thigh muscles. Look straight ahead, not down.

OWN IT: Hold for three minutes.

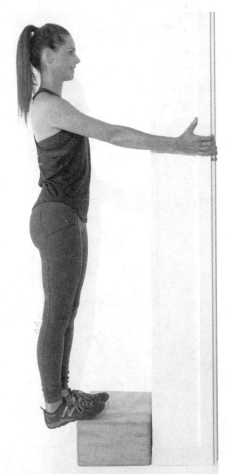

The Menu for Hips/Pelvis
(with Pain)

Short Foot......................................142

Hanging..143

Cats and Dogs................................144

Static Back....................................145

Hooklying Rocking Chair...............146

Unilateral Supine Femur Rotations ... 147

Pelvic Tilts 148

Static Extension.............................149

Cats and Dogs................................150

Air Bench......................................151

Short Foot

KNOW IT: Mimics proper foot and ankle movement during gait and starts to take away compensations in the load joints.

DO IT: Stand with your feet hip-width apart. Bring your right foot forward so that your right heel is in line with the toes of the left foot. Make sure both feet are pointing absolutely straight, and make sure your weight is evenly distributed in both feet. Bend your knees. In this position, lift the toes of the right foot up off the floor. Try to spread your toes apart as you pull them off the floor. Do not let the ball of the foot lift off the floor, lift only the toes. Next, press the toes into the floor without lifting the heel. Try to keep your toes elongated as you push down into the floor (don't curl your toes!). The arch of your foot will produce this motion, and you will feel the arch push upward when done correctly. Repeat on the other side, with the left foot in front.

OWN IT: Do three sets of ten repetitions on each side.

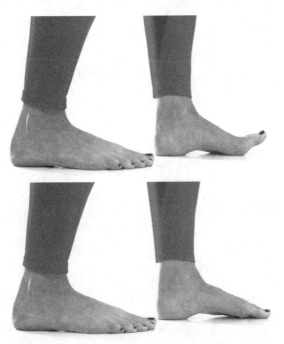

Hanging

KNOW IT: Elongates the muscles along the posterior side of the body, which often become tight and imbalanced from a lifestyle with too much sitting.

DO IT: Stand with your feet hip-width apart and pointed straight ahead. Bend over to touch your toes and hang, allowing the shoulders to relax. Drop your head and try to concentrate on relaxing your upper back. Keep your thighs tight and do not bend your knees or bounce. Keep your hips in line with your knees and ankles (don't stick your butt out behind you). If your hands don't reach the ground, let your arms hang loosely and allow gravity to slowly pull you closer to the ground. If your hands touch the ground, place your palms down with your fingers extended and allow gravity to slowly flatten your hands against the ground.

OWN IT: Hold for one minute.

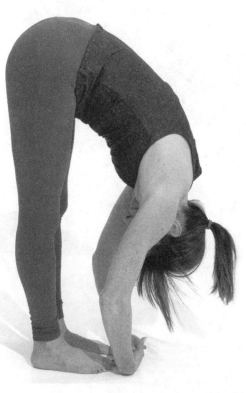

Cats and Dogs

KNOW IT: Works the hips, spine, shoulders, and neck in coordinated flexion-extension.

DO IT: Get down on the floor on your hands and knees. Make sure your knees are aligned with your hips, and your wrists with your shoulders. Your legs should be parallel with each other, and your feet relaxed with your toes pointed. Make sure your weight is distributed evenly. Smoothly round your back upward as your head tucks under to create a curve that runs from your butt to your neck (this is the cat with the arched back). Smoothly sway back down while bringing your head up and arching the back in the opposite direction (this is the gimme-a-treat dog). Try to initiate the movement with your pelvis. Make the two moves flow continuously back and forth rather than keeping them distinct and choppy.

OWN IT: Do one set of ten.

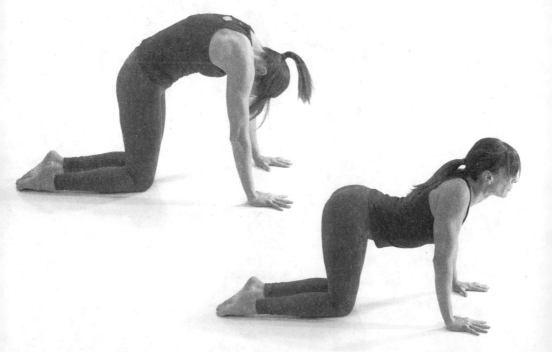

Static Back

KNOW IT: Settles your hips and back, releasing the compensating muscles that interfere with balance and functional movement.

DO IT: Lie on your back with both legs bent at right angles on a chair or block. Your hips should also be at ninety-degree angles. Rest your arms on the floor outstretched at forty-five-degree angles, with your palms up. Let your back settle into the floor, and breathe from your diaphragm (that is, do stomach breathing). Keep your abs relaxed (an easy test is to see if your stomach is rising and falling with each breath).

OWN IT: Hold this position for five minutes.

Hooklying Rocking Chair

KNOW IT: Improves range of motion in the ankle and coordinates the movement of the entire lower extremity.

DO IT: Lie on your back with your knees bent and your feet flat on the floor, pointed straight ahead. Your arms should be out to the sides at forty-five-degree angles, palms up. Place a pillow or block between your knees and keep light pressure against it. Keep your upper body relaxed. Roll both feet forward onto the ball of each foot (raising the heels off the ground). Keep your big toe engaged with the floor as you do so. Then roll both feet back onto the heel of each foot (raising the toes off the ground and pulling the foot back toward the shin). Keep gentle pressure against the block throughout the motion.

OWN IT: Do three sets of ten repetitions.

Unilateral Supine Femur Rotations

KNOW IT: Increases femur rotation and coordinates action of the major movers in the hips, pelvis, and lumbar spine.

DO IT: Lie on your back with your knees bent, arms out to the sides at forty-five degree angles with the palms facing up. Straighten one leg while keeping the other leg bent. On the straight leg, tighten your thigh and pull your toes back and hold. Rotate your leg and foot in and out, with the hip muscles initiating the movement. Do not rotate just the foot; the entire leg should be moving in and out while keeping the thigh tight and toes pulled back. Be sure to relax your upper body.

OWN IT: Do two sets of ten repetitions for each leg.

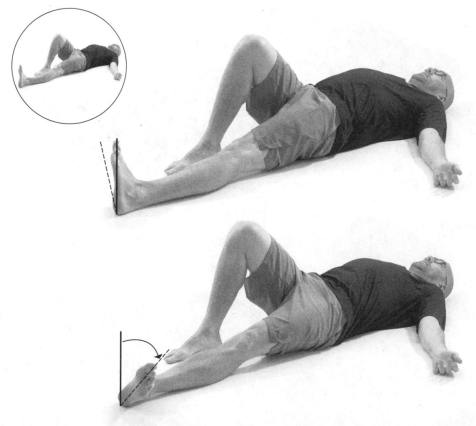

Pelvic Tilts

KNOW IT: Coordinates movement of the lower spine and pelvis.

DO IT: Lie on your back with your knees bent, feet flat on the floor, and arms out to the sides at ninety-degree angles. Roll your hips toward your torso to flatten your lower back into the floor. Do not lift your hips off the floor. Then roll your hips away to make your lower back arch off the floor, creating a space between the floor and your back. Do these rolls in a smooth and continuous motion, flattening your back into the floor and rolling the lower back off the floor by changing the tilt of your pelvis.

OWN IT: Do one set of ten repetitions.

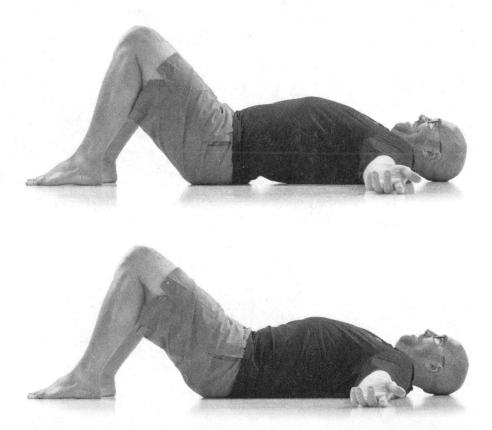

Static Extension

KNOW IT: Improves pelvic and spine imbalance to improve load joint function.

DO IT: Kneel on a block or ottoman with your hands on the floor. Shift your hips forward six to eight inches so that your hips are slightly in front of your knees. Work your hands out in front of you until your hands are directly under your shoulders. Let your back and head drop toward the floor and your shoulder blades come together. Relax your abs. Try to tilt your butt toward the ceiling and notice the pronounced arch in your lower back.

OWN IT: Hold for one or two minutes.

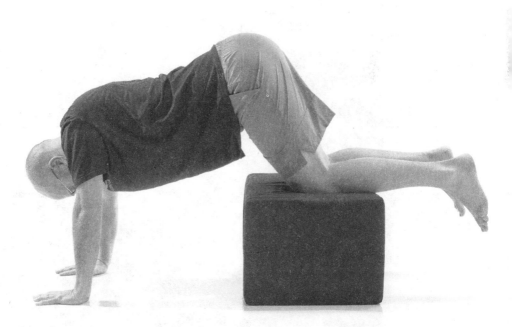

Cats and Dogs

KNOW IT: Works the hips, spine, shoulders, and neck in coordinated flexion-extension.

DO IT: Get down on the floor on your hands and knees. Make sure your knees are aligned with your hips, and your wrists with your shoulders. Your legs should be parallel with each other, and your feet relaxed with your toes pointed. Make sure your weight is distributed evenly. Smoothly round your back upward as your head tucks under to create a curve that runs from your butt to your neck (this is the cat with the arched back). Smoothly sway back down while bringing your head up and arching the back in the opposite direction (this is the gimme-a-treat dog). Try to initiate the movement with your pelvis. Make the two moves flow continuously back and forth rather than keeping them distinct and choppy.

OWN IT: Do one set of ten.

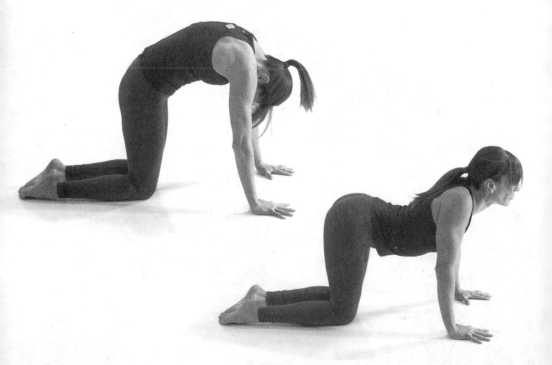

Air Bench

KNOW IT: Puts the hips, knees, and ankles simultaneously into flexion while they are under load.

DO IT: Stand with your back to a wall, and press your hips and the small of your back into the wall while walking your feet forward and sliding into a sitting position. Stop just before your hips reach a ninety-degree angle. Your knees should also be close to a ninety-degree angle, but your ankles should be just slightly forward of your knees. **Note:** If you feel pain in your knees, raise your body up the wall to relieve the pressure. Make sure your lower back is pressed against the wall and keep it pressed against the wall throughout the exercise. You should feel your quadriceps working along the top of the thigh.

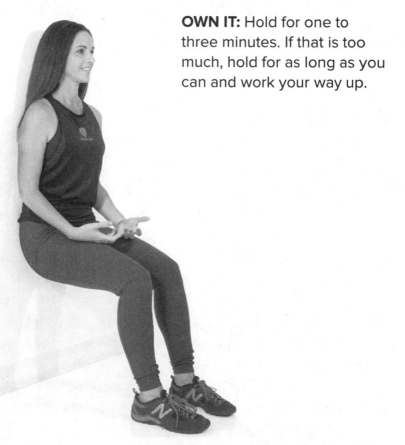

OWN IT: Hold for one to three minutes. If that is too much, hold for as long as you can and work your way up.

9

The Spine: Our Backbone of Function

Humans, unlike almost all other mammals, are designed to be bipeds. We are designed to move about the world on two limbs. The structure of our spine plays an enormous role in that two-legged existence, and, unsurprisingly, no other animal has anything quite like it. The human spine consists of vertebrae stacked one on top of the other. This is different from the spinal structure of most mammals, where the vertebrae are lined up one in front on the other. But what really sets us apart when it comes to form and function is our S-curve.

We have twenty-four vertebrae, which can be divided into three unique sections—the lumbar (lower back) spine, the

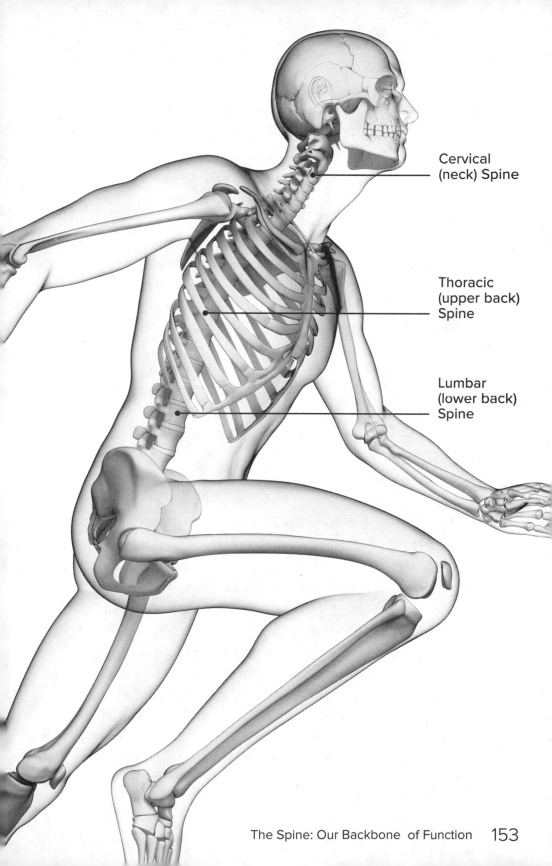

Cervical
(neck) Spine

Thoracic
(upper back)
Spine

Lumbar
(lower back)
Spine

thoracic (upper back) spine, and the cervical (neck) spine. Each section of our spine forms a unique curve. When viewed from the side, the thoracic spine resembles a C, and the lumbar and cervical curves mirror a backward C. Stacked together, the characteristic S-shape of the human spine appears.

Our spine acts like a highway, carrying information between the upper and lower body, with each curve managing information for a different part of the body. The cervical spine is responsible for head movement. The thoracic spine is responsible for movement of the torso and upper extremities. The lumbar spine is responsible for movement of the lower extremities. These unique curves work together to allow for more independent movement of our torso, extremities, and head.

Our S-curve perfectly balances the need for rigidity to stay upright with the need for flexibility to facilitate movement. We are capable of bending from front to back and side to side. We can rotate almost 180 degrees in either direction. And we can do all this while stabilizing the weight of our body in an upright position. No other animal even comes close to that kind of movement versatility.

Often, the easiest way to recognize the value of something is to take it away and see what changes. When it comes to our S-curve, this is perhaps best illustrated by a gorilla walking on its hind legs. Gorillas have a C-shaped spine and lack the mobility of our pelvis. As a result, gorillas take small steps and rock their weight from side to side to stay balanced and upright. These movements require a lot of energy, which is why gorillas only walk on two legs for short periods of time.

Our spinal curves prevent us from falling over by keeping the weight of the upper body centered over our mobile pelvis. We can take longer strides without losing our balance. Our mobile pelvis allows us to walk forward without the wasted energy of shifting our weight from side to side, making us much more efficient at upright ambulation.

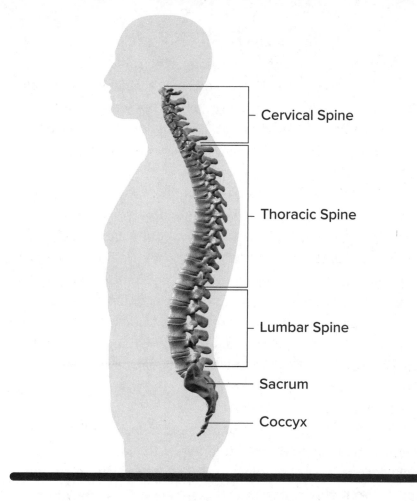

Cervical Spine

Thoracic Spine

Lumbar Spine

Sacrum

Coccyx

Spoiler alert: We are not immune from having to walk like gorillas. After all, we share 98 percent of our DNA with them, so we are more alike than different. We can lose the S-curve of our spine and the mobility of our pelvis. Without them, we start shuffling and rocking just like apes.

Gravity Wars

Our body is an antigravity machine. The drive shaft of that machine is the spine—its unique shape allows us to pull off our extraordinary balancing act. Muscles are essential to not only retain the spine's shape but also to hold it erect. Inactive, atrophied, and compensating muscles alter our lumbar, thoracic, and cervical curves. The muscles around the spine don't go all at once. Rather, it occurs gradually, as the body gets less and less stimuli from the environment. Our magical S diminishes, taking with it the spine's flexibility, load-bearing strength, and shock-absorbing capacity.

Confronted with an unstable spine, the body has one last-resort mechanism for utilizing what little power remains in atrophying muscles: it throws them into contraction. But the contracting muscles cannot defy gravity by holding the spine in place with sheer strength alone. The spine simply has too many moving parts. As the overworked muscles fatigue, the body grudgingly allows more and more flexion. But this too is a very finite tactic. Flex too far forward and the body becomes the victim of gravity's relentless pull. When the spine reaches the edge of this limit, desperate to remain upright, it quite literally freezes in place.

Let's get a clearer picture of the sequence. You climb into your 4x4 and head for home, determined to make the journey safely despite the ongoing blizzard. The road is icy, and a deer jumps in front of your truck. You hit the brakes, and they lock. You swing the steering wheel to the right and to the left, trying to prevent a skid. The truck fishtails wildly. That's what's happening with the muscles when our spine is out of balance. The compensating muscles, like a steering wheel, yank on the spine in a desperate attempt to keep it semimobile and reasonably upright. But the spine can't win under those circumstances. Short of total paralysis or rigor mortis, there is no escaping motion. The body must move. As the dysfunctional body moves, even a little, it wrings out the intended function of the bones, muscles, ligaments, tendons, and cartilage of the torso.

The simplest, most effective solution to back pain is based on a pure cause-and-effect relationship. Go after the muscles,

Fixed Flexion

You can feel how muscles sculpt your own back by sitting on the edge of a desk chair. Keep your feet flat on the floor, hip-width apart. Now, reach around with your right or left hand and place it on the small of the back, just above the waist. What do you feel? If you are like most people, the answer is, "Nothing much—a back." But you should notice immediately a pronounced concavity or arch—the lumbar curve. There is no missing it when it's there. If you have any doubt, it's not there.

Keep your hand on the small of your back. Slowly pull your head back and shoulders together without tightening the stomach muscles. Create some tension between the shoulder blades and within the upper back. Notice a change? There should be a more prominent lumbar curve. Now settle back into a natural position. You'll feel the arch straighten and disappear while the head sinks and the shoulders round forward. As this happens, the lumbar spine moves to the posterior along with the hips. The back is going into flexion. Sit upright again, and as the lumbar curve returns to your back, you will feel your hips rotate forward and the muscles on either side of your lower back engage. This is the position of the back in extension.

Muscles that don't move soon become muscles that cannot move. When we sit all day, with our backs and hips locked in flexion, the muscles that would normally bring our spine and pelvis back into extension become weak and inflexible. Spend enough time fixed in flexion and the body will slowly lose its ability to move into extension.

not the spine. Sure, there may be damage to the spine or its components—a herniated disc, nerve impingement, degenerative joints—but most back pain is caused by ongoing muscle imbalance. Put a stop to that dysfunction and the pain will subside. I have seen it happen literally thousands of times.

Danger—Sharp Thoracic Curve Ahead

The thoracic spine is designed with stability in mind. The vertebrae in this section are flanked on either side by rib bones, forming a protective cage around our vital organs and assisting with respiration. While the heart, the lungs, the liver, and the kidneys all receive added protection from this bony cage, its stiff, sturdy structure inherently limits the mobility of the thoracic spine. The cervical spine and lumbar spine are free-roaming, unrestricted by a surrounding bony cage, and intended to play a larger role in mobility.

If the lumbar or cervical spine starts to lose its mobility because of imbalance, weakness, or dysfunction, the thoracic back does its very best to pick up the slack. It's a trade-off that comes with a substantial price. The body is somewhat top-heavy to begin with. As the thoracic spine flexes to make up for lost mobility, it pulls our torso forward. The head and shoulders follow, and gravity gains even more traction. The opposing muscles of extension, rotation, and lateral movement tighten in reaction, working overtime to hold the imbalanced upper body erect. But it is a losing battle. These muscles are intended to allow movement in a variety of directions, but now thrown into contraction to hold the body upright, the only available movement that remains is more flexion. More flexion, more gravity, more tightness. More everything except function.

The thoracic back is truly a master of disguise. Thoracic

Scoliosis

Scoliosis most often affects adolescents experiencing sudden growth spurts. At puberty, the muscles and their intended functions may have a difficult time keeping up with the burgeoning skeletal structure. This is particularly true when the young person changes his or her established patterns of behavior, which is exactly what those entering their teenage years tend to do. Teenagers go from books to basketball and monkey bars to mascara in a flash. When such change coincides with a growth spurt, there is a drastic modification in the demand that is being put on the musculoskeletal system.

As the muscles struggle to adapt, imbalances in strength can occur from side to side. Form follows function. The stronger muscles pull the spine with more force than the weaker muscles can match. There is an unbalanced pull, and the spine begins to curve to the side. Scoliosis can be treated with a program of balanced muscular training. Reintroduce proper function, and the form of the spine will follow.

back issues tend to masquerade as rotator cuff, shoulder, and neck problems. Thoracic tightness gives way to achy shoulders and neck stiffness. Individuals complain of burning between the shoulder blades or trouble turning the head from side to side or lifting it up or down. But there are some tell-tale signs of thoracic back dysfunction. Head position is one. As the thoracic spine tries to compensate for lost mobility, it pulls the head and shoulders forward. A head that rests forward of the shoulders is a flashing red warning light for thoracic back issues. Repetitive shoulder shrugs and shakes signal a classic, but largely futile, effort to loosen up tight muscles. Thoracic imbalance leaves the shoulders and the head hanging in midair. Restoring balance is the only way to reestablish the intended structural support from the other load joints and ease the strain on the thoracic back and surrounding muscles.

Disc Risk

Herniated discs. Slipped discs. Bulging discs. If you have back pain, you have probably heard these terms tossed around. Full disclosure—each of these terms means the same thing and refers to an injury to the intravertebral disc.

In between each of our bony vertebrae sits an intravertebral disc. These discs behave like springy foam, acting as shock absorbers and buffers to prevent the bony vertebrae from colliding and grinding against one another during movement. The structure of the disc is similar to a jelly doughnut—the outer ring is rigid and holds the foamy center in place. Think of the center foam as a round marble that sits right in the center of the spine. As the vertebrae twist and turn, ascend, and descend, the marble of foam is centrally stationed to absorb and distribute force. As it is compressed, it pushes out equally in all directions against the rigid outer ring.

When the curve of the spine changes, the marble of spongy foam shifts away from the center of the disc. Now, when the marble is compressed, one edge of the disc has to buffer a much greater force than the other. If that pressure is great enough, the rigid outer ring can no longer hold the spongy foam in place. The center jelly starts to leak or bulge out of the intravertebral disc, often compressing nearby nerves and causing pain.

Herniated discs are often treated surgically, either by remov-

Disc Dicussion

The firm outer ring of the intervertebral disc is known as the annulus fibrosus. This more rigid structure acts to hold the spongy center, known as the nucleus pulposus, within the disc. The nucleus pulposus is like a spongy marble that can be compressed to help absorb and distribute force.

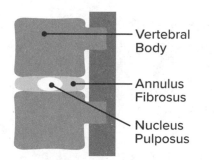

Vertebral Body

Annulus Fibrosus

Nucleus Pulposus

NORMAL INTERVERTEBRAL DISC

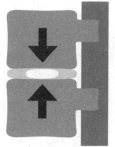

COMPRESSED INTERVERTEBRAL DISC

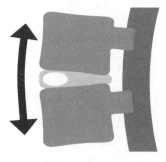

HYPEREXTENSION

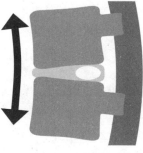

FLEXION

When the "marble" is located in the center of the intervertebral disc, the force of its compression is distributed evenly in all directions against the annulus fibrosus. If the position of the spine changes, the position of the marble follows suit. Instead of being located centrally, the marble shifts to one side or the other within the intervertebral disc. Now, when it is compressed, one side of the annulus fibrosus must withstand a much greater force than the other, increasing the likelihood of injury.

ing part of the injured disc or by removing the disc entirely and fusing the adjacent vertebrae to keep the spine stable. This removes the pressure on nearby nerves and tissue and can provide pain relief, but it does nothing to address the reason *why* the disc herniated to begin with. The abnormal stress on the intravertebral disc has not changed, leaving it vulnerable to recurrent herniations. And, in the case of spinal fusions, the now immobile joint places even more stress on the surrounding intravertebral discs, placing them at great risk for injury. It is no wonder patients frequently suffer subsequent disc herniations after spine surgery.

My hope is that by now you know there is an alternative. Get the foamy marble back into the center of the intravertebral disc by restoring our intended spinal curves. By shifting the entire vertebral column back into alignment, the nearby nerves are given back the much-needed space necessary for pain relief. And the removal of all the excess strain on the intravertebral disc allows the herniation to heal naturally.

Muscle Spasms

Anyone who has suffered through a back spasm knows how excruciating it can be. Back pain can have a can't-breathe, can't-move, all-consuming urgency. Back spasms result from muscles contracting uncontrollably. In short, this unwillingness to relax means that any opposing motion triggers pain that literally stops you in your tracks.

Often muscle spasms are a protective response to an injury. Our immediate response to musculoskeletal pain is to stop what we are doing and rest. The body intuitively responds the same way, activating muscles to protect and rest an injured area by redirecting pressure and stress elsewhere. But back spasms can also be a Hail Mary attempt to compensate for underlying imbalance and dysfunction.

S or C?

We have all seen the consequences of losing our S-curve—even if we did not realize it at the time. The characteristic hunchback appearance when the spine more closely resembles a C rather than an S? Those people characteristically have a shuffling, shortened stride. Their mobility is profoundly decreased. Not only that—the hunchback requires much more effort from his muscles to stay upright. This decreases the additional work these muscles are capable of doing in response to our ever-changing, unpredictable environment. The result is an inherently less stable biped who is more prone to balance loss and falls. Similarly, these changes place abnormal strain on the muscles, bones, and joints, increasing the likelihood that these structures break down and cause injury and pain.

Take a Breather

Pain and mobility are good reasons to invest in restoring your S-curve, but here is another. Our thoracic curve affects lung function. When the thoracic curve becomes more pronounced (think hunchback), the lungs' ability to expand decreases. Excessive thoracic curvature weakens respiratory muscles and restricts your ability to take a full, deep breath.

When the integrity of our spinal curve is lost, the spine is at the mercy of gravity—and gravity is merciless. Without the flexibility needed for balance, the muscles around the spine resort to continual contraction. That continuous contraction does the exhausting work of keeping the body upright in the absence of balance, but the cost is often catastrophic pain.

Contracting muscles are complicated. In the ultimate sense, the choice between permanent contraction and permanent relaxation is a choice between life and death. For a muscle, work is required to prevent atrophy. That said, no muscle will tolerate an unrelenting demand for work without complaint.

Our saving grace comes from restoring our S-curve. That, and that alone, will reduce the effort required to stay upright and reduce the strain on the bones, joints, and muscles. Muscles are fast learners. Given the chance to relax without tumbling over or worsening an injury, even the angriest muscles will breathe a sigh of relief.

The Secret to Six-Pack Abs

Want a six-pack? Get an S-curve. I am not kidding. Many of my athletes say they get "free abs" from doing their menu. There is actually a lot of truth in that message. When dysfunction sets in, the abdominal muscles frequently go on a permanent vacation. The abs are designed to play a major role in posture and movement, but they can only do that when the pelvis and spine are aligned. You can do sit-ups until your face turns blue, but if your spine and pelvis inhibit proper abdominal muscle function, that six-pack will remain elusive.

Water Your Spine

Staying hydrated and getting quality sleep have more to do with back health than you might expect. The cushion at the center of an intravertebral disc is composed of 85 percent water. That water concentration is critical to its shock-absorbing function. Research shows that movement throughout the day drops that water concentration by about 20 percent. Lying down at night removes the pressure from the intravertebral disc and allows the lost water to flow back into the center cushion. The disc also obtains nutrients through this continuous loss and replenishment of fluid. Dehydration can limit this critical function, leaving the disc compressed, and compromising its ability to buffer force.

The Menu for Backs

(Lumbar Pain/ Herniated Discs)

Sitting Knee Pillow Squeezes 167

Static Back with Knee Pillow
Squeezes 168

Modified Floor Block...................... 169

Static Extension............................. 170

Air Bench.. 171

Static Back...................................... 172

Lying Supine.................................... 173

Air Bench.. 174

Sitting Knee Pillow Squeezes

KNOW IT: Strengthens hip adductors and reduces disparity by placing balanced and systematic demand on the pelvis.

DO IT: Sit on the edge of a chair or bench, and arch your back by rolling your hips forward. Pull your shoulders back, and make sure your knees are in alignment with your hips. Point your feet straight ahead. Your feet should be directly beneath your knees. Relax your stomach muscles (let them hang). Place a pillow between your knees. Using your inner thighs, squeeze the pillow and release it gently. You may need to fold the pillow to give it thickness. The pillow should be thick enough that your knees stay aligned with your hips as you squeeze. Your feet should stay parallel to each other (and don't let your stomach or upper back engage in the movement).

OWN IT: Do three sets of ten repetitions.

Static Back with Knee Pillow Squeezes

KNOW IT: Helps to balance pelvis and torso to allow proper movement of the hip and proper rotation of the femur.

DO IT: Lie on your back with both legs bent at right angles on a chair or block. Your hips should also be at ninety-degree angles. Rest your arms on the floor outstretched at forty-five-degree angles, with your palms up. Let your back settle into the floor, and breathe from your diaphragm (that is, do stomach breathing). Keep your abs relaxed (an easy test is to see if your stomach is rising/falling with each breath). Hold for three minutes. Place a pillow between your knees. Using your inner thighs, squeeze the pillow and release, applying pressure evenly on either side of the block. Your feet should remain parallel to each other.

OWN IT: Hold static back for three minutes. Then do three sets of ten repetitions of knee pillow squeezes.

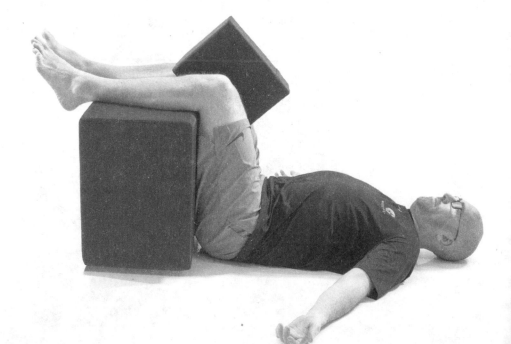

Modified Floor Block

KNOW IT: Coordinates shoulder, torso, and pelvic movement.

DO IT: Lie on your stomach with your forehead on the floor, your feet pigeon-toed (toes pointed, ankles relaxed), and your butt relaxed. Rest your forearms on six-inch-high blocks (lower if this causes discomfort) with your wrists relaxed and your hands dangling over the blocks' front edge. Your arms should extend at ninety degrees from the shoulder and should bend ninety degrees at the elbow. Make sure your shoulders are level from right to left. Breathe deeply and relax the upper body. Don't press your arms into the blocks. Let your stomach muscles relax.

OWN IT: Hold for six minutes.

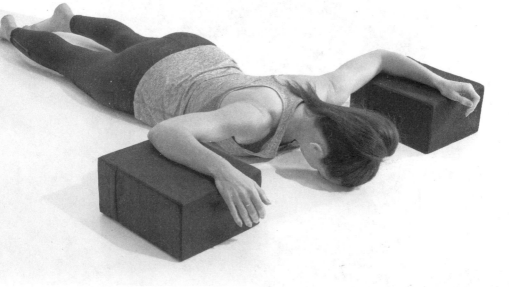

Static Extension

KNOW IT: Improves pelvic and spine imbalance to improve load joint function.

DO IT: Kneel on a block or ottoman with your hands on the floor. Shift your hips forward six to eight inches so that your hips are slightly in front of your knees. Work your hands out in front of you until your hands are directly under your shoulders. Let your back and head drop toward the floor and your shoulder blades come together. Relax your abs. Try to tilt your butt toward the ceiling and notice the pronounced arch in your lower back.

OWN IT: Hold for one or two minutes.

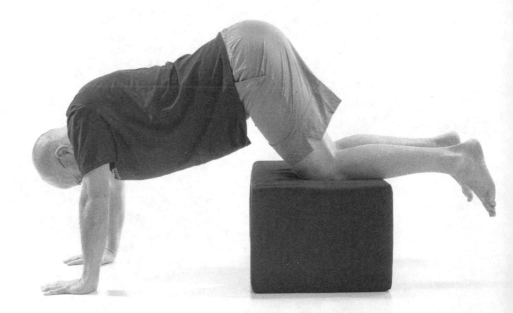

Air Bench

KNOW IT: Puts the hips, knees, and ankles simultaneously into flexion while they are under load.

DO IT: Stand with your back to a wall, and press your hips and the small of your back into the wall while walking your feet forward and sliding into a sitting position. Stop just before your hips reach a ninety-degree angle. Your knees should also be close to a ninety-degree angle, but your ankles should be just slightly forward of your knees. **Note:** If you feel pain in your knees, raise your body up the wall to relieve the pressure. Make sure your lower back is pressed against the wall and keep it pressed against the wall throughout the exercise. You should feel your quadriceps working along the top of the thigh.

OWN IT: Hold for one to three minutes. If that is too much, hold for as long as you can and work your way up.

Static Back

KNOW IT: Settles your hips and back, releasing the compensating muscles that interfere with balance and functional movement.

DO IT: Lie on your back with both legs bent at right angles on a chair or block. Your hips should also be at ninety-degree angles. Rest your arms on the floor outstretched at forty-five-degree angles, with your palms up. Let your back settle into the floor, and breathe from your diaphragm (that is, do stomach breathing). Keep your abs relaxed (an easy test is to see if your stomach is rising and falling with each breath).

OWN IT: Hold this position for five minutes.

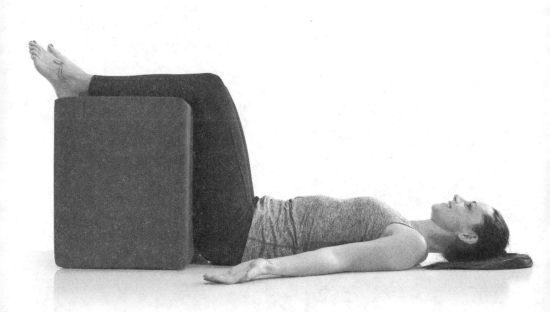

Lying Supine

KNOW IT: Helps to improve joint position and balance throughout the kinetic chain.

DO IT: Lie on your back with both legs straight and flat on the floor. Place a pillow or small block between your ankles/feet. Flex your toes back toward your hips, bending at the ankle joint. Keep gentle pressure along the block with the insides of your feet. Try to keep your upper body relaxed, with arms at forty-five-degree angles to your body, palms up. Tighten the thigh muscles.

OWN IT: Hold for three to five minutes.

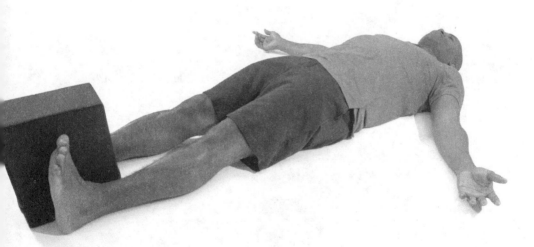

Air Bench

KNOW IT: Puts the hips, knees, and ankles simultaneously into flexion while they are under load.

DO IT: Stand with your back to a wall, and press your hips and the small of your back into the wall while walking your feet forward and sliding into a sitting position. Stop just before your hips reach a ninety-degree angle. Your knees should also be close to a ninety-degree angle, but your ankles should be just slightly forward of your knees. **Note:** If you feel pain in your knees, raise your body up the wall to relieve the pressure. Make sure your lower back is pressed against the wall and keep it pressed against the wall throughout the exercise. You should feel your quadriceps working along the top of the thigh.

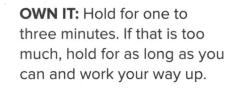

OWN IT: Hold for one to three minutes. If that is too much, hold for as long as you can and work your way up.

The Menu for Backs
(Thoracic Back Pain)

Static Back....................................... 176

Reverse Presses............................... 177

Pullovers... 178

Floor Block 179

Static Extension.............................. 180

Squat 181

Static Back

KNOW IT: Settles your hips and back, releasing the compensating muscles that interfere with balance and functional movement.

DO IT: Lie on your back with both legs bent at right angles on a chair or block. Your hips should also be at ninety-degree angles. Rest your arms on the floor outstretched at forty-five-degree angles, with your palms up. Let your back settle into the floor, and breathe from your diaphragm (that is, do stomach breathing). Keep your abs relaxed (an easy test is to see if your stomach is rising and falling with each breath).

OWN IT: Hold this position for five minutes.

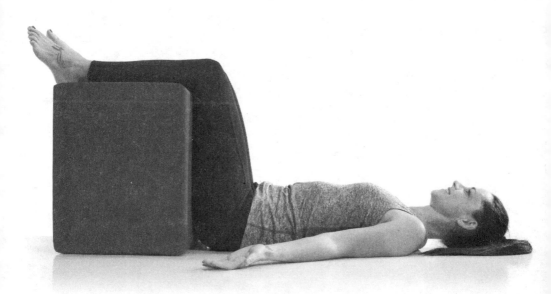

Reverse Presses

KNOW IT: Improves scapula mobility and reduces compensation in the thoracic spine.

DO IT: From the Static Back position, with your legs propped at ninety degrees, place your elbows straight out from your shoulders. Bend your elbows and form a loose fist with each hand. Point the knuckles up to the ceiling. Your wrist, forearm, and hand should be in a straight line. Press your elbows and the back of your arms straight down into the floor. Don't jerk. Concentrate on allowing the shoulder blades to come together. Hold for a moment and release.

OWN IT: Do fifteen times, three sets.

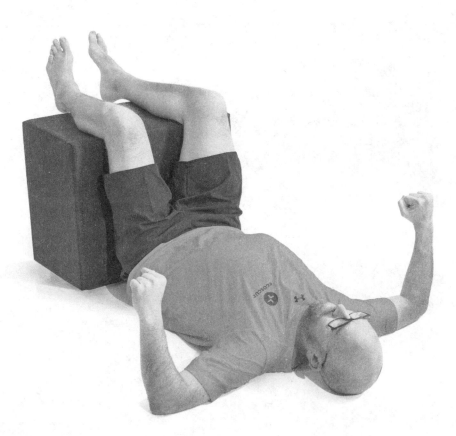

Pullovers

KNOW IT: Improves shoulder mobility and reduces compensation in the thoracic spine.

DO IT: From the Static Back position, clasp your hands together tightly with your fingers interlaced. Extend your elbows straight to the ceiling. Continuing to hold both arms straight, bring them back over your head, either to the floor or as far as they will go without bending. Return to the starting position with your arms extended straight to the ceiling. Relax your abdominal muscles, and don't rush.

OWN IT: Do fifteen times, three sets.

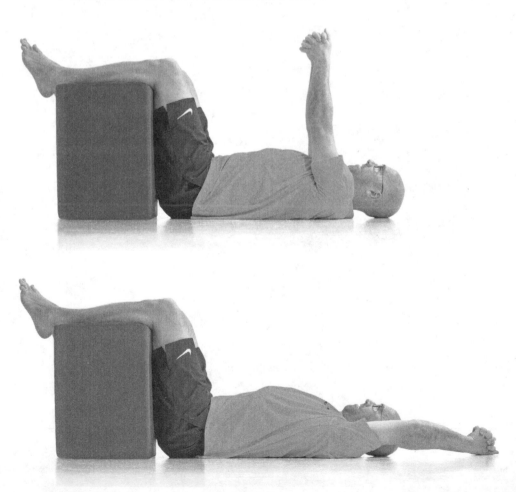

Floor Block

KNOW IT: Coordinates movement of the humerus and scapula and helps to balance the torso and spine.

DO IT: Lie on your stomach, facedown and arms over your head, with your elbows straight and feet pigeon-toed. Rest your forearms on six-inch blocks. Place your hands in a golfer's grip with your fingers curled, knuckles flexed, and thumbs extended, and point your thumbs toward the ceiling. Place your forehead on the floor and keep your neck, shoulder, butt, and stomach relaxed. Move your arms outward, away from your body, and continuously try to get more range throughout the exercise. Initiate the movement from your shoulders, not your elbows. Hold for one minute, then repeat with your arms at 10 o'clock and 2, and then again at 9 o'clock and 3.

Use the "golfer's grip," see page 81 for details.

OWN IT: Hold for one minute in each position.

Static Extension

KNOW IT: Improves pelvic and spine imbalance to improve load joint function.

DO IT: Kneel on a block or ottoman with your hands on the floor. Shift your hips forward six to eight inches so that your hips are slightly in front of your knees. Work your hands out in front of you until your hands are directly under your shoulders. Let your back and head drop toward the floor and your shoulder blades come together. Relax your abs. Try to tilt your butt toward the ceiling and notice the pronounced arch in your lower back.

OWN IT: Hold for one or two minutes.

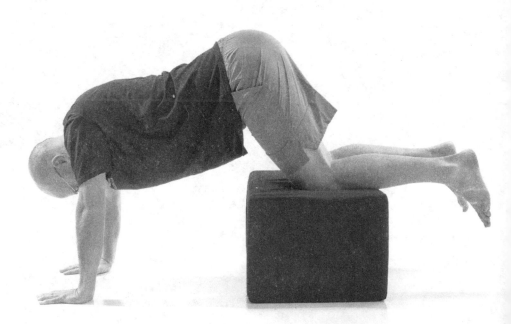

Squat

KNOW IT: Properly recruits the major movers of the lower body and pelvis while reducing upper-body compensation.

DO IT: Holding on to a rail, pole, or doorknob for support, bend your knees and arch your lower back. Keep your torso straight and your shoulders back. Lower your body so your knees and hips are parallel. Your arms should be straight. Your knees should be directly above your feet, which should be pointed straight ahead. Your torso should remain vertical throughout. Try not to bend your torso forward.

OWN IT: Hold for one to two minutes.

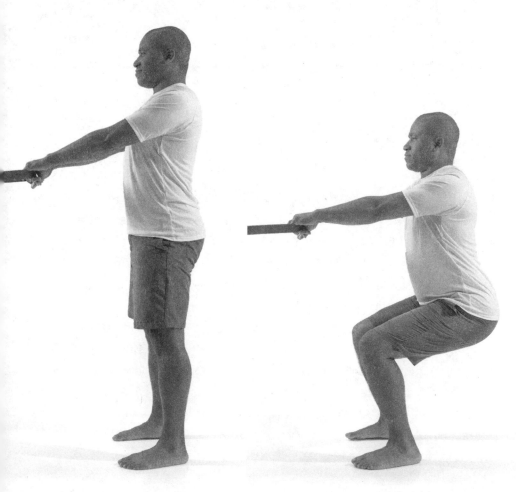

10

The Shoulders: The Mobility King

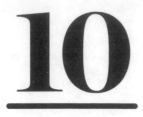

Free, unrestricted use of our upper extremities is probably the most advantageous by-product of walking about on two feet. Intellectual insight aside, your dog cannot help you carry groceries inside. He cannot paint the house, swing a golf club, or even refill his own water bowl (okay, you might be able to train him to try, but I am willing to bet more water ends up on your floor than in your dog's mouth). Even if he had hands with the versatility of ours, his upper extremities would be occupied with walking around instead of free to accomplish other tasks. We have the freedom to use our hands and upper extremities exclusively as a tool to explore and interact with our environment. No other species has that advantage.

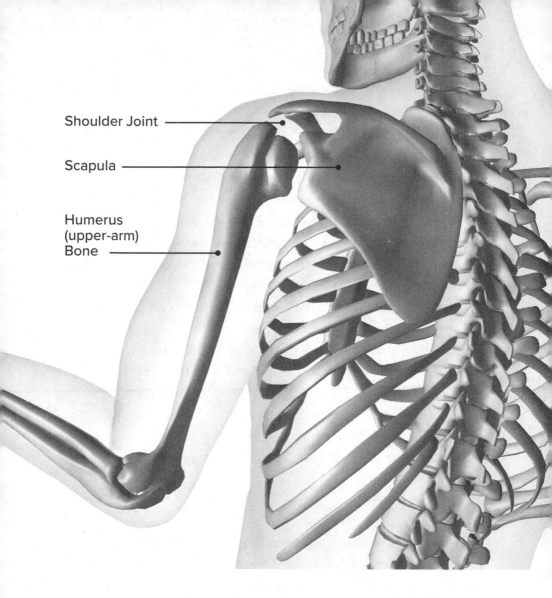

Shoulder Joint

Scapula

Humerus
(upper-arm)
Bone

Four-legged animals split weight-bearing responsibilities across all their extremities. In humans, the shoulders do play a load-bearing role when it comes to supporting the head and neck, but the majority of the responsibility for weight-bearing falls to the lower extremities. Without the continual need to support the weight of our body, the upper extremity is free to move unanchored to the ground. Our shoulder is the starting point of this unique upper-extremity function.

The shoulder connects the upper extremity to the body via

a ball-and-socket joint. Much like the hip, it is designed to allow an extraordinary amount of movement. In fact, when it comes to range of motion, the shoulder tops every other joint in the body. The socket of the hip (the pelvis) is relatively fixed, capable of important but small movements. On the other hand, the shoulder socket (the scapula) is very mobile. That mobile platform allows us to raise our arms above our head; to reach forward, backward, and out to the side; and to twist our upper extremities with ease. The hip is slightly less mobile than the shoulder but more stable. The shoulder wins out in the mobility contest but sacrifices some stability in doing so.

Immense mobility requires a lot of support. That support comes from the surrounding muscles and ligaments. The four muscles collectively known as the rotator cuff are responsible for positioning the head of the humerus (the bone of the upper arm) in the shoulder joint and holding the top of the humerus close to the scapula to stabilize the joint. That is a big job, and unfortunately our motionless existence has set the rotator cuff up as a notoriously problematic supporting actor.

Boxed In

The daily demand on our shoulder joint is on a precipitous decline. Our ancestors climbed, crawled, hoisted logs and buckets of water overhead, and shot bows and arrows. In our modern world, shoulder motion has been squeezed into an invisible three-by-four-foot box that hangs in midair directly in front of us, covering an area from roughly the midthighs to the armpits. We do little outside of this box, which means we fail to routinely use more than 50 percent of our shoulder's function. Muscles require use to maintain function. We aren't *using it,* so we end up *losing it*.

Wrestle a suitcase out of an overhead bin? Rake leaves? Hit a tennis ball? These jobs are no big deal—we have the muscles,

Opposing Sides

Mobility and stability have an inverse relationship. If you look at an X-ray of the hip, the ball and socket have a fair amount of overlap. The top of the femur actually rests inside the depression in the pelvic bone. That inherently limits some of the joint's mobility and increases the hip's stability. A shoulder X-ray has a different appearance. The arm bone (the humerus) sits in a slightly depressed area of the shoulder blade (the scapula). But there is less overlap between the two bones when compared to the hip joint. This frees up some extra mobility in the shoulder but also decreases the joint's inherent stability.

SHOULDER JOINT

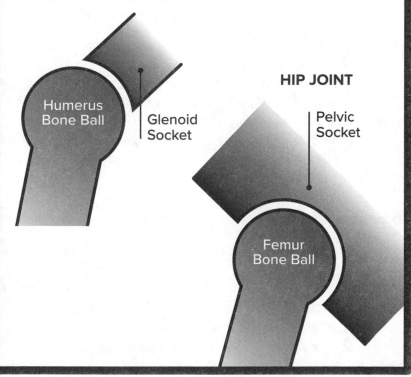

Humerus
Bone Ball

Glenoid
Socket

HIP JOINT

Pelvic
Socket

Femur
Bone Ball

When was the last time you . . .

☐ Got down on the floor?

☐ Hung by your hands?

☐ Crawled on your hands and knees?

☐ Reached behind you, to the left and the right?

☐ Climbed over an object (a fence or large rock)?

☐ Climbed under an object (a porch or low-hanging tree)?

☐ Put both hands on the top of your head?

☐ Balanced on one foot?

☐ Balanced on one foot while elevated above the ground (atop a stump, stool, or bench)?

☐ Stood on your tippy-toes?

☐ Danced?

If you go through the list and answer each question deliberately—not with "it's been a while" but with an actual length of time—I think you will be shocked. There will be activities that you haven't done in years—maybe decades. Not because they are dangerous, difficult, or physically tasking. But because climbing out of modern society's box of routine movement requires deliberate action. For most of us, our modern movements—no matter how repetitively or energetically we perform them—are not sufficient to

bones, and joints to do all of them easily and safely. But these tasks fall outside our shoulder's modern movement box. We foolishly left our shoulder functions outside, like tricycles and roller skates abandoned in the grass of the front yard to rust away. Now, when we move outside that safe box, we hurt.

Modern motion is so limited and based so much on re-

maintain musculoskeletal health.

All of us can perform each of the activities on the above list. The human body comes equipped with the capability to do them all. Yet few of us do. Time-lapse photography would show that the box of modern shoulder movement is shrinking. As the head comes forward and the spine takes on the shape of a C, shoulder movements become more and more restricted. Episodic shoulder pain is a warning: Stay inside the box! Chronic shoulder pain tells us that the steadily shrinking box has now become too small to accommodate even the most limited, routine movement. We end up living in a box because we cannot live pain free outside of it.

Musculoskeletal functions that are not regularly used become inaccessible. And while we might act surprised when we ask the shoulders to do something seemingly simple and get pain instead, deep down, we are far from shocked. "I should have known better than to . . ." Fill in the blank with your injury-ridden activity of choice. The phrase is common and demonstrates that we are at least subconsciously aware of our restricted function even before pain makes it blaringly obvious. Restoring function is the only true cure for the pain, but the real magic comes from reconnecting with our sub-conscious awareness that something is off-kilter. If we learn to feel imbalance before pain sets in, we are well on our way to living pain free.

petitive patterns that we have eliminated the shoulder almost entirely from our routine activities. Interestingly, few people suspect that their tightness or pain might have something to do with the fact that before we encountered that paintbrush, tennis racket, or suitcase, we had not been outside the shoulder's modern movement box in months, or even years. We seem to forget that muscles that are not used turn into muscles that cannot be used (at least not without consequences).

Reach for the Sky

Few people reach directly over their heads more than a couple of times per year and even less bear any weight in that position. Yet all of us have a carefully calibrated mechanism to do just that. Unused muscles become weak. The body's function is designed around balance, and weak muscles (even infrequently used weak muscles) disrupt that balance.

Our motionless lower body and spine potentiate the problem. Hips and back muscles weakened by endless hours of sitting leave the shoulders and head rounded forward. The muscles that allow us to raise our arms above our head are the same muscles that help keep our shoulders back and our heads up. With compounding imbalance and dysfunction, the body is forced to start compensating. And while those compensations are adequate for a time, the end result is devastatingly simple. The continual stress and strain of abnormal demand on the muscles, bones, and joints inevitably leads to injury and pain. The only way to fix it—or better yet, prevent it—is to restore our musculoskeletal balance.

Fooorrre

In many ways, the dynamics of the shoulder joint closely mirror a golf ball sitting on a tee. When the golf ball is centered over the tee, the ball stays balanced on the tee without any additional effort. If you place the golf ball on the tee a little too far forward or off to one side, the ball will wobble. You will either catch and redirect it or watch as it falls to the ground. The rotator cuff has a very similar job when it comes to the shoulder joint.

Rotator Cuff

The bones of the shoulder resemble a golf ball balanced on a golf tee. When balanced, the rotator cuff has to do minimal work to keep the golf ball (the humerus) balanced on the tee (the scapula). When the shoulder falls out of balance, the rotator cuff muscles must do extra work to stabilize the joint, and keep the golf ball from falling off the tee.

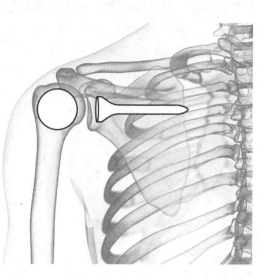

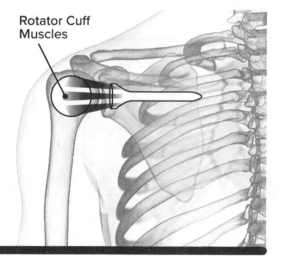

Rotator Cuff Muscles

When the joint is positioned properly and aligned with the rest of the load joints, minimal effort is required from the rotator cuff to keep the joint balanced. Muscle imbalance changes the resting position of the joints. A shift in any direction changes the balance of demand on the individual muscles that make up the rotator cuff. Some muscles become overworked and strained, prone to injury because of a lack of recovery and rest.

Others become underused and weak, prone to injury because of inadequate strength to meet unexpected demands. Either way, the rotator cuff muscles are forced to continuously catch an unbalanced golf ball to prevent it from falling off its tee. Our motionless existence is increasingly making muscular imbalance the norm instead of the exception. No wonder rotator cuff injuries are so frustratingly common.

Strength in Triangles

The hips and the shoulders have an intricate relationship that plays a large role in dictating our overall ability to move.

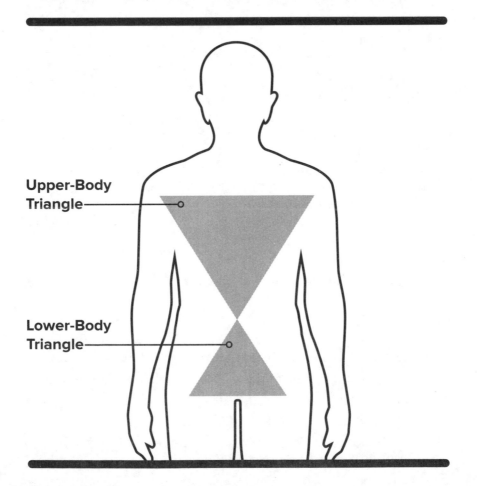

Upper-Body Triangle

Lower-Body Triangle

Imagine the human trunk as being composed of two triangles balanced tip to tip. The base of one triangle runs across the hips with the top point resting at the bottom of the thoracic spine. This can be thought of as the lower-body triangle. The base of the other triangle runs across the shoulders, pointing down and resting on the tip of the first triangle. This is the upper-body triangle. When the body is balanced, the upper-body and lower-body triangles meet point to point and resemble a balanced hourglass, able to stay upright with minimal effort.

When we spend so much of our lives sitting, the position of the hips inevitably changes, taking on the shape of the chair and shifting backward. The tip of the lower-body triangle follows. The upper body must adjust to keep the triangles connected. The shoulders roll forward, shifting the base of the upper-body triangle forward. The tip of the upper-body triangle points back, maintaining the connection with the lower body. But now, instead of a vertically balanced hourglass that can stay upright without assistance, we have a V-shaped hourglass that wants to fall backward. Our muscles must do extra work to fight that tendency, work that is misaligned and imbalanced. The body moves and responds as a unit. We feel pain and suffer injuries in isolation, but the abnormal stress and strain that caused these problems can be alleviated only with solutions that restore connection.

Function Fix

Want to see how readily the shoulders rely on the other load joints? Stand against a wall, with your heels touching the base of the wall. To begin, stand with your feet pointed out like a duck. Take note of your shoulder position. What parts of your shoulders are making contact with the wall?

Now, stand pigeon-toed, pointing your feet in, and relax your stomach muscles. Tighten your thigh muscles (take note if it is harder to fully straighten your legs in this position). Notice how much more of your shoulder is in contact with the wall? You also probably noticed that you are standing taller. Standing pigeon-toed merely duplicates what your muscles are supposed to do naturally and automatically, creating a more balanced state between your load joints and spine.

Self-Test

Want to see how muscles we don't use become muscles we can't use? Stay seated. Roll your shoulders forward and let your back curve into an exaggerated C-shape (modern society's weak posture). Raise your arms out in front of you as high as you can. Now raise them out to the side as high as you can. Can't get very far, right? Now pull your shoulders back and straighten your spine (think good, strong posture). Now repeat the two tests. Yup—big difference.

The Menu for Shoulders
(with Pain)

Standing Wall with Block 194

Sitting Knee Pillow Squeezes 195

Sitting Heel Raises with Block 196

Three-Position Toe Raises 197

Wall Stork 198

Static Back 199

Progressive Supine Groin 200

Cats and Dogs 201

Air Bench 202

Standing Wall with Block

KNOW IT: Promotes proper positioning of all load joints.

DO IT: Stand at a wall with your heels, hips, and upper back against the wall. Place a small block or pillow between your knees. Apply gentle pressure, just enough to hold the pillow in place; do not push into it. It's okay if your head is not against the wall. Stand in a relaxed position and let your head rest naturally. With enough time, your head will move back on its own; don't force it. Relax your stomach and your arms and allow your body to adjust to this new position. Keep your thighs tight so that your knees are locked in a straight, or extended, position. Remember to keep your feet pointed straight ahead and your stomach relaxed throughout.

OWN IT: Hold for six to eight minutes.

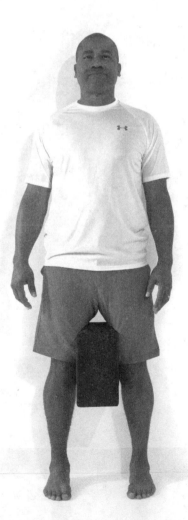

Do supersets of the following three exercises—
that is, do ten repetitions of the first, then ten repetitions
of the second, then ten of the third.
Then repeat the cycle for a total of three times through.

Sitting Knee Pillow Squeezes

KNOW IT: Strengthens hip adductors and reduces disparity by placing balanced and systematic demand on the pelvis.

DO IT: Sit on the edge of a chair or bench, and arch your back by rolling your hips forward. Pull your shoulders back, and make sure your knees are in alignment with your hips. Point your feet straight ahead. Your feet should be directly beneath your knees. Relax your stomach muscles (let them hang). Place a pillow between your knees. Using your inner thighs, squeeze the pillow and release it gently. You may need to fold the pillow to give it thickness. The pillow should be thick enough that your knees stay aligned with your hips as you squeeze. Your feet should stay parallel to each other (and don't let your stomach or upper back engage in the movement).

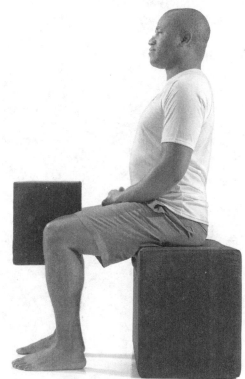

OWN IT:
Do three sets of ten repetitions.

Sitting Heel Raises with Block

KNOW IT: Helps to coordinate movement of the entire lower extremity.

DO IT: Sit on the edge of a chair or bench, and arch your lower back by rolling your hips forward. Place a pillow or foam block between your knees and gently squeeze the block. Your toes should remain pointed straight ahead and your big toe should remain the center point of contact with the floor throughout the motion. Raise your heels. Don't push off your toes; instead, use your hip flexor muscles (imagine your toes are resting on eggshells to keep them relaxed).

OWN IT: Do three sets of ten repetitions.

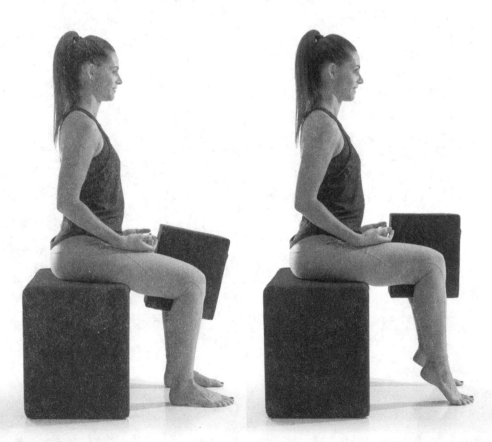

Three-Position Toe Raises

KNOW IT: Coordinates and balances the motion of the load joints with various rotational demands on the lower extremity.

DO IT: Near a closed door or wall, stand with your feet straight ahead, hip-width apart, with your weight distributed evenly between them. Turn your toes out to forty-five degrees. Slowly raise yourself up onto your toes and then lower yourself back to the ground so your feet are once again flat on the floor. Make sure to keep pressure between your big toe and the ground throughout the entire motion. Keep your weight evenly distributed between both feet. Do ten repetitions. Now bring your feet parallel with your toes pointing forward. Do ten repetitions. Now angle your toes inward about twenty degrees and do ten repetitions. Make sure your heels remain wider than your toes as you go up and down (you will likely notice they want to move in as you come down; don't let them).

OWN IT: Do two sets of ten toe raises in each position.

Wall Stork

KNOW IT: Strengthens independent movement of the hips and balances the pelvis, torso, and lower extremity.

DO IT: Stand with your back against the wall with your feet hip-width apart, pointing straight ahead. Your heels, hips, and upper back should be against the wall. Place one foot on a chair in front of you. Your knee should be bent to ninety degrees, thigh parallel to the floor. Make sure that your foot is pointed straight. Do not allow the standing leg to bend or shift to the side. (Your hip, knee, and ankle should stay in a straight line.) Tighten the thigh muscle of the straight leg. Keep the shoulder and hip on the bent-leg side flat against the wall.

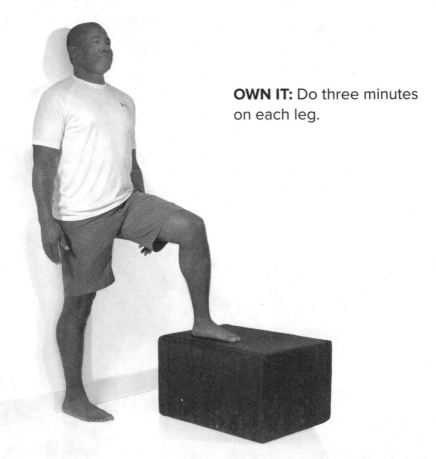

OWN IT: Do three minutes on each leg.

Static Back

KNOW IT: Settles your hips and back, releasing the compensating muscles that interfere with balance and functional movement.

DO IT: Lie on your back with both legs bent at right angles on a chair or block. Your hips should also be at ninety-degree angles. Rest your arms on the floor outstretched at forty-five-degree angles, with your palms up. Let your back settle into the floor, and breathe from your diaphragm (that is, do stomach breathing). Keep your abs relaxed (an easy test is to see if your stomach is rising and falling with each breath).

OWN IT: Hold this position for five minutes.

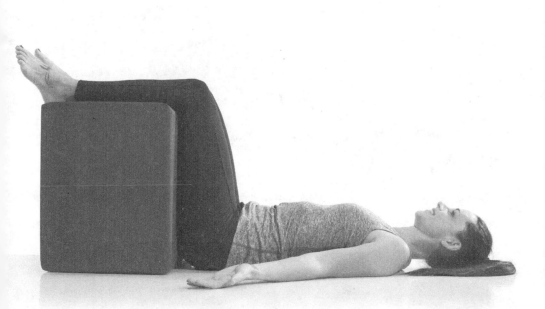

Progressive Supine Groin

KNOW IT: Allows for proper flexion and extension of the leg while reducing compensating side-to-side and rotational motions.

DO IT: Lie on your back with one leg resting on a block or chair, your knee bent at a ninety-degree angle, while the other leg is extended on a small stepladder, a stack of books, or something of a similar height (so that your back and hips are flat on the floor). Prop the outside of your foot on the extended leg to prevent it from rolling out. Let the leg rest at this top level for three to five minutes. Ideally, your lower back should come to rest flat against the floor before moving on. Lower your extended foot about five to eight inches and repeat for three to five minutes. Continue to progressively lower your extended foot five to eight inches at a time until your foot is resting against the floor. Again, let the leg rest along the floor until your lower back rests flat on the floor. Don't try to flatten your back.
Let it happen naturally.

OWN IT: Hold each position for three minutes, and repeat on the opposite side.

These images depict Progressive Supine Groin using the Egoscue tower, a tool specifically designed for the exercise. You can complete the exercise without the tower as described above.

Cats and Dogs

KNOW IT: Works the hips, spine, shoulders, and neck in coordinated flexion-extension.

DO IT: Get down on the floor on your hands and knees. Make sure your knees are aligned with your hips, and your wrists with your shoulders. Your legs should be parallel with each other, and your feet relaxed with your toes pointed. Make sure your weight is distributed evenly. Smoothly round your back upward as your head tucks under to create a curve that runs from your butt to your neck (this is the cat with the arched back). Smoothly sway back down while bringing your head up and arching the back in the opposite direction (this is the gimme-a-treat dog). Try to initiate the movement with your pelvis. Make the two moves flow continuously back and forth rather than keeping them distinct and choppy.

OWN IT: Do one set of ten.

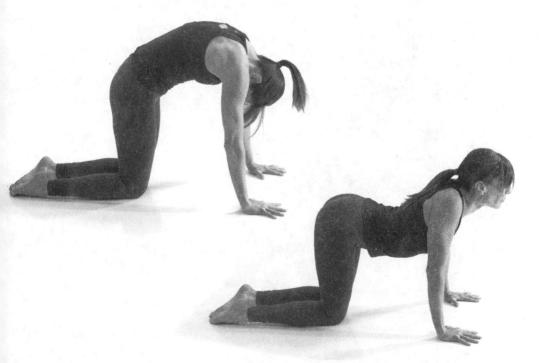

Air Bench

KNOW IT: Puts the hips, knees, and ankles simultaneously into flexion while they are under load.

DO IT: Stand with your back to a wall, and press your hips and the small of your back into the wall while walking your feet forward and sliding into a sitting position. Stop just before your hips reach a ninety-degree angle. Your knees should also be close to a ninety-degree angle, but your ankles should be just slightly forward of your knees. **Note:** If you feel pain in your knees, raise your body up the wall to relieve the pressure. Make sure your lower back is pressed against the wall and keep it pressed against the wall throughout the exercise. You should feel your quadriceps working along the top of the thigh.

OWN IT: Hold for one to three minutes. If that is too much, hold for as long as you can and work your way up.

The Menu for Shoulders

(No Pain, but Motion Restriction)

Sitting Knee Pillow Squeezes 204

Static Extension 205

Sitting Floor 206

Seated Arm Circles 207

Squat 208

Cats and Dogs 209

Sitting Knee Pillow Squeezes

KNOW IT: Strengthens hip adductors and reduces disparity by placing balanced and systematic demand on the pelvis.

DO IT: Sit on the edge of a chair or bench, and arch your back by rolling your hips forward. Pull your shoulders back, and make sure your knees are in alignment with your hips. Point your feet straight ahead. Your feet should be directly beneath your knees. Relax your stomach muscles (let them hang). Place a pillow between your knees. Using your inner thighs, squeeze the pillow and release it gently. You may need to fold the pillow to give it thickness. The pillow should be thick enough that your knees stay aligned with your hips as you squeeze. Your feet should stay parallel to each other (and don't let your stomach or upper back engage in the movement).

OWN IT:
Do three sets of ten repetitions.

Static Extension

KNOW IT: Improves pelvic and spine imbalance to improve load joint function.

DO IT: Kneel on a block or ottoman with your hands on the floor. Shift your hips forward six to eight inches so that your hips are slightly in front of your knees. Work your hands out in front of you until your hands are directly under your shoulders. Let your back and head drop toward the floor and your shoulder blades come together. Relax your abs. Try to tilt your butt toward the ceiling and notice the pronounced arch in your lower back.

OWN IT: Hold for one or two minutes.

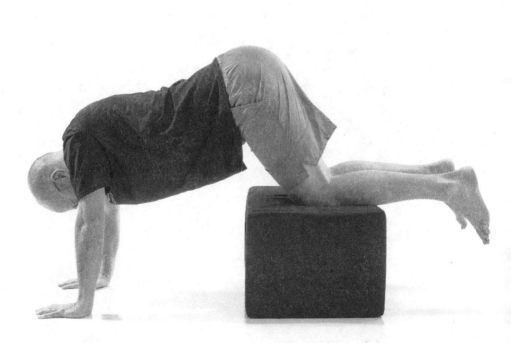

Sitting Floor

KNOW IT: Promotes thoracic extension and upper-body balance while eliminating rotation in your lower extremities.

DO IT: Sit against a wall with your legs straight out in front of you. Your butt and upper back should be against the wall the entire time. Squeeze your shoulder blades together and hold. Do not lift the shoulders; squeeze them back and down. Tighten your thighs and flex the feet so that your toes are pointing back toward you. Relax your hands, palms up, and rest them on your thighs. Look straight ahead. Keep your shoulders back, your thighs tight, and your feet flexed throughout the exercise.

OWN IT: Hold for four to six minutes.

Seated Arm Circles

KNOW IT: Strengthens the muscles of the upper back and shoulders, and balances the top of the kinetic chain and pelvis.

DO IT: Sit on a chair or bench with your head up, feet squared, and arms at your sides. Keep your feet pointed straight ahead. Put your hands in the golfer's grip with your fingers curled, knuckles flexed, and thumbs extended. Raise your arms out to the sides, keeping your elbows straight, palms down, and thumbs pointing forward. Lift your arms until they are level with your shoulders. If one shoulder wants to wobble forward or pop up, lower both until they stay level. Now squeeze your shoulder blades together slightly, and rotate your arms forward in a six-inch-diameter circle. Then, reverse the circle by turning your palms up and thumbs back. Always make the circles in the direction that the thumb is pointing. Don't let your arms drop as you do the circles.

OWN IT: Do fifty with your palms down and fifty with your palms up.

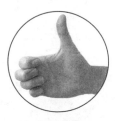

Use the "golfer's grip," see page 81 for details.

Squat

KNOW IT: Properly recruits the major movers of the lower body and pelvis while reducing upper-body compensation.

DO IT: Holding on to a rail, pole, or doorknob for support, bend your knees and arch your lower back. Keep your torso straight and your shoulders back. Lower your body so your knees and hips are parallel. Your arms should be straight. Your knees should be directly above your feet, which should be pointed straight ahead. Your torso should remain vertical throughout. Try not to bend your torso forward.

OWN IT: Hold for one to two minutes.

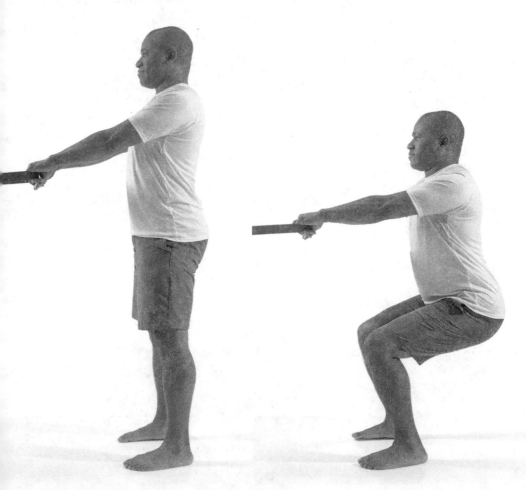

Cats and Dogs

KNOW IT: Works the hips, spine, shoulders, and neck in coordinated flexion-extension.

DO IT: Get down on the floor on your hands and knees. Make sure your knees are aligned with your hips, and your wrists with your shoulders. Your legs should be parallel with each other, and your feet relaxed with your toes pointed. Make sure your weight is distributed evenly. Smoothly round your back upward as your head tucks under to create a curve that runs from your butt to your neck (this is the cat with the arched back). Smoothly sway back down while bringing your head up and arching the back in the opposite direction (this is the gimme-a-treat dog). Try to initiate the movement with your pelvis. Make the two moves flow continuously back and forth rather than keeping them distinct and choppy.

OWN IT: Do one set of ten.

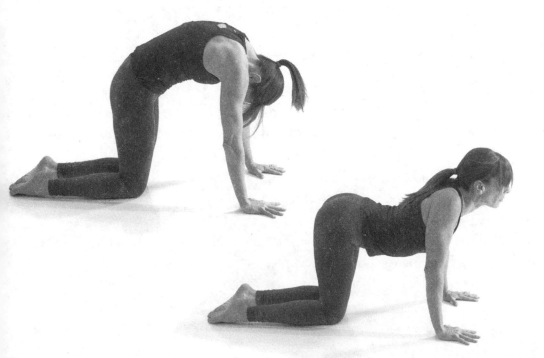

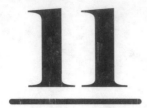

Head and Neck: The Crown of Balance

The head and neck occupy the most preeminent position in the anatomical hierarchy. Nothing else holds a higher position on our musculoskeletal totem pole. The head's significance is obvious. It houses the brain—the omnipotent conductor of our movements, memories, perceptions, emotions, and intellect. Given the brain's importance to everything human, the head is nothing short of a fortress, encasing our crown jewel in a house of protective bone. The top part of our characteristic S-curve—the cervical spine—runs from the shoulders to the base of the skull. If we consider the brain to be human royalty,

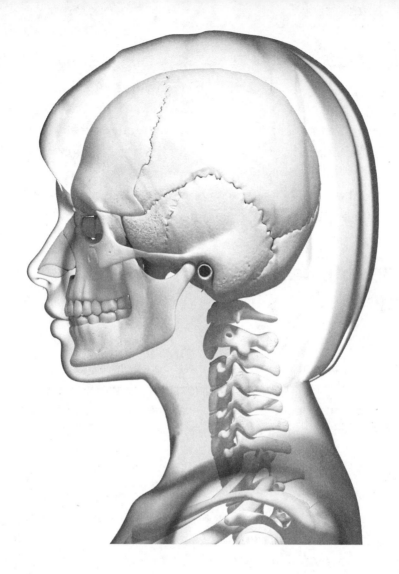

the neck quite literally provides a throne upon which the head can safely rest.

As the musculoskeletal system ascends past the upper back, its load-bearing capacity becomes more and more dependent on a stable foundation of muscles, bones, and joints. The lumbar and thoracic spine are supported by the torso, hips, and shoulders, surrounded by major muscle groups on either side. Above the shoulders, an intricate balancing act must occur. The cervical spine extends upward as the sole anchor and base of support for the head.

We are born with the bony structure of the neck, but its characteristic curve is developed by learning to lift and move the head against the force of gravity. That, and that alone, is the purpose of the cervical curve: to hold the head vertically while allowing for independent movement of the head. Our cervical curve allows us to freely twist, turn, and bend at the neck, which increases the amount of head movement we can achieve without relying on simultaneous movement of our torso.

From Heads Up to Hunkered Down

Walking about the world on two legs, humans have an evolutionary advantage when it comes to our line of sight. We can see farther simply because our heads are higher (relative to our body size). Of course, that advantage requires that we look out, not down. But in modern society, we are looking down—a lot.

We already know that the average person spends three hours a day staring at their cellphone screen. Have you ever seen someone hold their phone at eye level? Nope—we hold them within our little safety box of shoulder movement and look down. We spend hours sitting and looking down at textbooks, computer screens, and newspapers. Looking down is not in and of itself the problem. After all, looking down is one of the many versatile movements in which our head and neck are designed to partake. But looking down all the time disrupts the delicate balance of the muscles responsible for holding the head upright. Once imbalance sets in, it is only a matter of time until we feel the other shoe painfully drop.

The head is designed to rest atop the neck aligned vertically with the shoulders, hips, knees, and ankles. When the joints are aligned in this manner, the spine will have its characteristic

Around the Horn

Humans are developing a new skeletal trait—hornlike spikes on the back of the skull. Research shows this trait is more common in younger generations. The bony growth occurs at the bottom of the skull and is attributed to the increasing prevalence of forward head position. When the head sits in a forward position, weight is shifted away from the vertebrae and increasingly onto the muscles of the neck. The bony growths in the connecting tendons and ligaments help to buffer this increased workload.

S-shape, and the work needed to hold the body (and the head) upright will be minimized. You can easily test this for yourself. The head weighs ten to twelve pounds. Find something with a similar weight and hold it directly above your head with your arm straight. Now move your arm three inches forward. Now six inches. It takes a lot more work to hold the weight out in front of your body than directly overhead.

Our modern lives of minimal motion, excessive sitting, and persistent downward gaze are distorting the spine's S-curve into a C. As we sit and our spine gradually conforms to the chair, our shoulders slump forward, bringing the head along for the ride. When we stare down, we bend the neck forward to shift our line of sight. With the head tilted forward, gravity literally has us by the nose. The muscles that would normally hold the head upright are forced to do more and more work to fight gravity's relentless downward pull. The body has great tolerance. But it does not have infinite tolerance. Pain is frequently the first message to alert us that we have exceeded the limits of the body's tolerance.

Future Shock—Dysfunctional Children

A few decades ago, a gawky teenager whose head was forward and whose shoulders slouched was probably showing signs of nothing more than a rapid growth spurt. Before long, the muscles would catch up, gaining the strength necessary to properly support the child's larger and heavier frame. Today, teenagers still undergo growth spurts, but now they occur in the context of an increasingly motionless environment. Gone are the days of playing outside until dark and performing manual chores in the yard. Kids today can most commonly be found sitting in front of a computer or television. That environment does not provide the stimulus necessary to awaken and strengthen the supporting musculoskeletal functions. The muscles never catch up to the growing skeleton. Thus, the head moves forward, not at sixty years old but at sixteen.

Once upon a time, our first lessons in musculoskeletal function were passed down from our parents. I used to routinely hear parents telling their children to stand or sit up straight. This was not just a platitude to make offspring appear more presentable. Forty years ago, we still had some sense of what musculoskeletal health *looked* like. C-shaped spines, slouched shoulders, and heads that tilted down were not signs of health, happiness, or prosperity. Today, we have become so accustomed to seeing heads out of position that we seldom even consciously recognize it.

Off Balance and Out of Whack

Aside from stressing out our neck muscles and placing abnormal strain on our bones and intervertebral discs, shifting the head's position throws off our entire sense of equilibrium. To maintain balance and navigate the world, we rely on three

Shift Work

Even a small forward shift of the head's position has an enormous impact on the amount of work the neck muscles must do to anchor the head in place. When the head is aligned and sitting directly above the other load joints, the neck muscles must do the work necessary to support ten to twelve pounds of weight. As the head moves forward and tilts down, the relative weight of the head increases. This means that the neck muscles are being asked to do more and more work to anchor the head in place. Even a small shift of one to two inches forward of our vertical line creates two to three times as much work for the neck muscles.

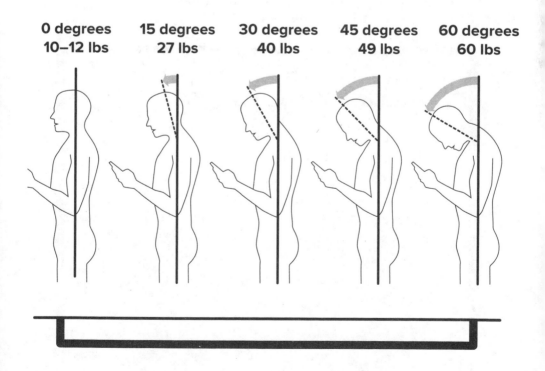

0 degrees
10–12 lbs

15 degrees
27 lbs

30 degrees
40 lbs

45 degrees
49 lbs

60 degrees
60 lbs

sources of information: proprioception, visual input, and vestibular input. Proprioception comes from our muscles and joints, providing information about where we are in space. Visual input comes from our eyes, seeing where we are in relationship to everything else. Vestibular input comes from the inner ear. Three fluid-filled tubes in the inner ear provide information about up-and-down, side-to-side, and tilting movements of the head relative to gravity.

When the head is tilted forward, the inner ear assumes the body is going downhill. Our eyes reflexively adjust for changes in head position to hold our field of vision steady. The eyes see the surface as flat and provide conflicting information to the brain. Vision is our most powerful sense, accounting for somewhere between 50 and 60 percent of our brain's processing power. When there is a conflict, vision wins. The eyes overpower the inner ear and we feel balanced. We aren't balanced, but the eyes win—for now.

Bouts of dizziness occur when the body starts to fatigue

Check Your Balance

Stand up straight and close your eyes. Stay that way until you start to sway. How long was it? Some people have to open their eyes after only ten to twenty seconds to prevent themselves from falling over. When the eyes are open, vision overrides the inner ear's balancing mechanism. Without vision, the inner ear takes over. A dysfunctional head position (tilted forward or leaning to one side) will immediately create sensations of being off balance.

from attempting to process the continuously conflicting signals it is getting from the eyes and the inner ears. The sheer burden of fighting a losing struggle against gravity in a state of misalignment exceeds the body's tolerance, and vertigo (dizziness) ensues. The ability to read terrain becomes difficult and chancy, and falls become a major hazard.

Vertical alignment is our best line of defense when it comes to preventing and treating debilitating bouts of dizziness. Similarly, it is also our best line of defense against unexpectedly losing our balance and falling over. When our three equilibrium systems are aligned, our balance commanders are cooperating instead of fighting against one another. "United we stand, divided we fall" is not just a political truth. It is very much biological.

Headaches

The world is full of headache sufferers. Many of them have undergone a battery of diagnostic tests and, all too often, all of them have come up blank. That is because the most frequent causes of headache will not show up on any of our fancy imaging or diagnostic tests. Sure, some life-threatening causes such as brain bleeds and tumors will show up, but thankfully these are zebras when it comes to headaches. (In medicine, a zebra is an unlikely diagnosis.) The most common causes—hunger, dehydration, stress, lack of sleep, lack of oxygen, muscle tension—will not.

It seems obvious to start with the most common causes and move toward the least common, but that is generally not the formula used by modern medicine. Before the era of instant answers, physicians almost always started with the most common cause of a problem. And you know what, many of their patients got better because common things are common. Today, technology makes it easy to jump straight to zebra hunting.

But unless you have a rare breed of stripes, odds are you will just end up frustrated, with a persistent headache, and without answers even after all that extensive testing.

The most common cause of headaches is muscle tension. Tense or overcontracted neck muscles are the culprit behind most headaches. The easiest solution—get your head out of its forward position and remove the continuous demand for extra work from your neck muscles. Lack of oxygen is another common cause. When the spine is C-shaped, with the shoulders rolled forward, the chest cavity is constricted and the amount of oxygen the diaphragm can pull in with each breath is reduced. Both of these culprits can easily be fixed with exercises that restore the spine's natural S-curve.

I am not knocking modern medicine. The body is complex, and not every headache can be treated by addressing musculoskeletal balance. But it is a simple place to start, and common things being common, the odds are forever in your favor.

Function and Flow

Most people never consider that posture has a direct impact on blood flow. An unstable, semi-collapsed musculoskeletal system cannot efficiently perform its role as an oxygen delivery pump. Sharp thoracic curves and rounded shoulders limit the expansion of the lungs and reduce the amount of oxygen that can be brought in with each breath, but the problem doesn't stop there. Research has shown that the rate of blood flow to the brain is influenced by the curve of the neck. Individuals with decreased or reversed cervical curves (like those whose head sits three inches forward of the shoulders) had significantly decreased flow through the large vessels that supply blood to the brain. When a curved pillow was placed underneath the neck to restore the cervical curve, there was a dramatic improvement in the rate of blood flow to the brain.

Pillow Fights

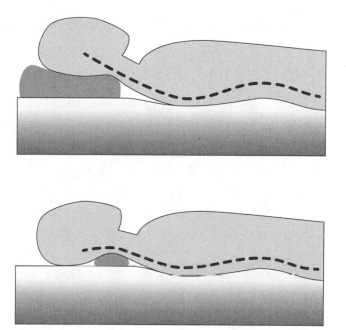

When we lose our cervical curve (top), the rate of blood flow through the large vessels in our neck decreases. Placing a pillow underneath the neck to restore the natural cervical curve (bottom) has been shown to increase the rate of flow through these vessels, increasing the amount of oxygen and nutrients reaching our brain.

Blood flow is critical when it comes to delivering fresh oxygen to our cells, and the brain is extremely sensitive to even relatively small fluctuations in oxygen availability. There is a growing body of evidence that links dementia, headaches, concussions, and traumatic brain injury with cerebral blood flow. And while there are plenty of things in life that we cannot control, the position of our head and neck is not one of those things. We can retrain our muscles to restore our cervical curve and improve our brain's oxygen lifeline in the process.

Concussion Crisis

Today's sports world is on a mission to decrease the pandemic of concussions occurring across all levels of competition. We are investing millions of dollars into custom helmets and diagnostic tools, and yet understanding why some hits cause concussions and others do not remains a challenge. What we do know is this—concussions are related to the amount of rotational acceleration the head (and brain) experience after an impact. And guess what—neck position matters. Even small changes in cervical spine position can increase rotational acceleration by more than 100 percent.

The Menu for Necks

(Cervical Spine/ Neck Herniations)

Standing Wall with Block.............. 222

Short Foot..................................... 223

Static Extension............................ 224

Hero's Pose.................................. 225

Sitting Knee Pillow Squeezes 226

Air Bench..................................... 227

Standing Wall with Block

KNOW IT: Promotes proper positioning of all load joints.

DO IT: Stand at a wall with your heels, hips, and upper back against the wall. Place a small block or pillow between your knees. Apply gentle pressure, just enough to hold the pillow in place; do not push into it. It's okay if your head is not against the wall. Stand in a relaxed position and let your head rest naturally. With enough time, your head will move back on its own; don't force it. Relax your stomach and your arms and allow your body to adjust to this new position. Keep your thighs tight so that your knees are locked in a straight, or extended, position. Remember to keep your feet pointed straight ahead and your stomach relaxed throughout.

OWN IT: Hold for six to eight minutes.

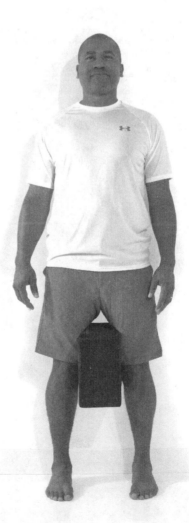

Short Foot

KNOW IT: Mimics proper foot and ankle movement during gait and starts to take away compensations in the load joints.

DO IT: Stand with your feet hip-width apart. Bring your right foot forward so that your right heel is in line with the toes of the left foot. Make sure both feet are pointing absolutely straight, and make sure your weight is evenly distributed in both feet. Bend your knees. In this position, lift the toes of the right foot up off the floor. Try to spread your toes apart as you pull them off the floor. Do not let the ball of the foot lift off the floor, lift only the toes. Next press the toes into the floor without lifting the heel. Try to keep your toes elongated as you push down into the floor (don't curl your toes!). The arch of your foot will produce this motion, and you will feel the arch push upward when done correctly. Repeat on the other side, with the left foot in front.

OWN IT: Do three sets of ten repetitions on each side.

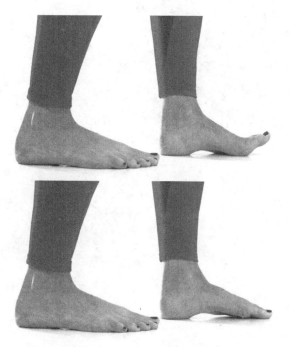

Static Extension

KNOW IT: Improves pelvic and spine imbalance to improve load joint function.

DO IT: Kneel on a block or ottoman with your hands on the floor. Shift your hips forward six to eight inches so that your hips are slightly in front of your knees. Work your hands out in front of you until your hands are directly under your shoulders. Let your back and head drop toward the floor and your shoulder blades come together. Relax your abs. Try to tilt your butt toward the ceiling and notice the pronounced arch in your lower back.

OWN IT: Hold for one or two minutes.

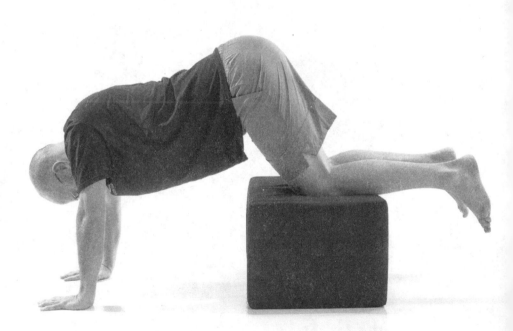

Hero's Pose

KNOW IT: Promotes symmetric pelvic and torso position.

DO IT: Kneel down with your knees and ankles together and sit on your heels. Your toes should be pointed so the tops of your feet and ankles are on the floor. If this is too difficult, place a pillow between your ankles and sit on that to raise your butt up from the ankle level. Relax your upper body as you roll your hips forward to arch your lower back. Keep your arms and upper back relaxed. Allow your shoulder blades to move "down and back," but don't force it. Let it happen naturally as you hold the position. Relax your abdominal muscles.

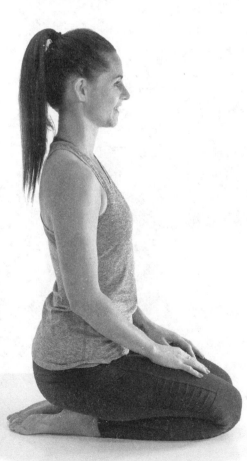

OWN IT: Hold for one minute.

Sitting Knee Pillow Squeezes

KNOW IT: Strengthens hip adductors and reduces disparity by placing balanced and systematic demand on the pelvis.

DO IT: Sit on the edge of a chair or bench, and arch your back by rolling your hips forward. Pull your shoulders back, and make sure your knees are in alignment with your hips. Point your feet straight ahead. Your feet should be directly beneath your knees. Relax your stomach muscles (let them hang). Place a pillow between your knees. Using your inner thighs, squeeze the pillow and release it gently. You may need to fold the pillow to give it thickness. The pillow should be thick enough that your knees stay aligned with your hips as you squeeze. Your feet should stay parallel to each other (and don't let your stomach or upper back engage in the movement).

OWN IT:
Do three sets of ten repetitions.

Air Bench

KNOW IT: Puts the hips, knees, and ankles simultaneously into flexion while they are under load.

DO IT: Stand with your back to a wall, and press your hips and the small of your back into the wall while walking your feet forward and sliding into a sitting position. Stop just before your hips reach a ninety-degree angle. Your knees should also be close to a ninety-degree angle, but your ankles should be just slightly forward of your knees. **Note:** If you feel pain in your knees, raise your body up the wall to relieve the pressure. Make sure your lower back is pressed against the wall and keep it pressed against the wall throughout the exercise. You should feel your quadriceps working along the top of the thigh.

OWN IT: Hold for one to three minutes. If that is too much, hold for as long as you can and work your way up.

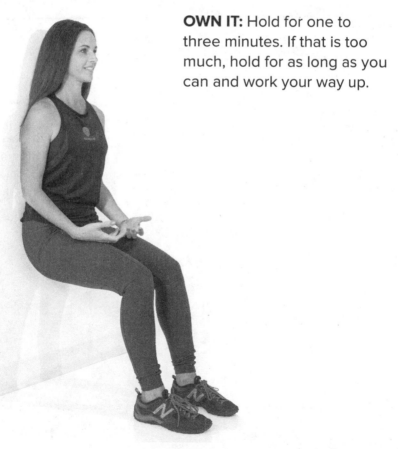

The Menu for Headaches

Standing Wall with Block.............. 229

Slant Board Ankle Sequence........ 230

Static Extension........................... 235

Static Back.................................... 236

Pullovers....................................... 237

Cats and Dogs.............................. 238

Standing Wall with Block

KNOW IT: Promotes proper positioning of all load joints.

DO IT: Stand at a wall with your heels, hips, and upper back against the wall. Place a small block or pillow between your knees. Apply gentle pressure, just enough to hold the pillow in place; do not push into it. It's okay if your head is not against the wall. Stand in a relaxed position and let your head rest naturally. With enough time, your head will move back on its own; don't force it. Relax your stomach and your arms and allow your body to adjust to this new position. Keep your thighs tight so that your knees are locked in a straight, or extended, position. Remember to keep your feet pointed straight ahead and your stomach relaxed throughout.

OWN IT: Hold for six to eight minutes.

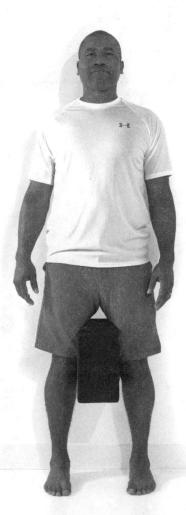

Slant Board Ankle Sequence

KNOW IT: Uses the ankle joint to strengthen the muscles of the pelvis, activating the hip flexor so that vertical posture facilitates dynamic tension from the front to the back of the body.

DO IT: Sit slouched on a chair and place your feet on a slant board so that your knees are at least two inches above your hip level. Place your feet hip-width apart and pointed straight ahead.

Positions 1 and 2 require the slant board to face you, so the feet are angled up.

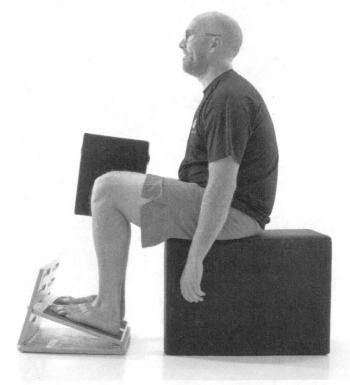

Position 1

Place a pillow between your knees and squeeze and re-lease it twenty times. After this initial set of squeezes/re-leases, squeeze the pillow and maintain constant pressure on the pillow for the following foot/ankle movements.

Using the muscles on the front side of your lower leg, lift the balls of your feet and toes up off the slant board so that only the heels are in contact. Return them to the slant board and repeat twenty times. Then, using the muscles on the back of your lower leg, push your heels up off the slant board so that only the balls of your feet and toes are in contact. Return your heels to the slant board and repeat twenty times. Keep continuous pressure between your big toe and the slant board as you raise your heel and go up onto your toes.

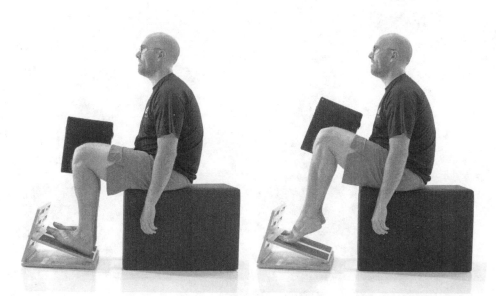

Position 2

Place a strap around your knees. Push your legs out against the strap and release it twenty times. After this initial set of pushouts and releases, push out against the strap and maintain constant pressure on the strap for the following foot/ankle movements.

Using the muscles on the front of your lower leg, lift the balls and toes of your feet up off the slant board so that only the heels are in contact. Return them to the slant board and repeat twenty times. Then, using the muscles on the back of your lower leg, push your heels up off the slant board so that only the balls of your feet and toes are in contact. Return your heels to the slant board and repeat twenty times. Keep continuous pressure between your big toe and the slant board as you raise your heel.

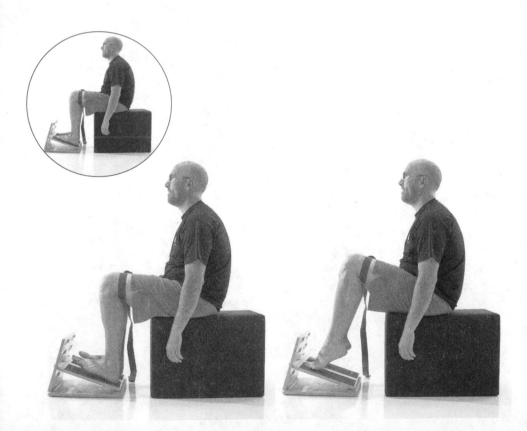

Position 3

Place a pillow between your knees and squeeze and release it twenty times. After this initial set of squeezes/releases, squeeze the pillow and maintain constant pressure on the pillow for the following foot/ankle movements.

Using the muscles on the back of your lower leg, push your heels up off the slant board so that only the balls of your feet and toes are in contact with the board. Return your heels to the slant board and repeat twenty times. Keep continuous pressure between your big toe and the slant board as you raise your heel and go up onto your toes. Then, using the muscles on the front side of the lower leg, lift the balls of your feet and toes up off the slant board so only your heels are in contact with the board. Return your toes to the slant board and repeat twenty times.

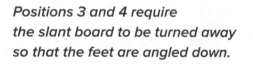

Positions 3 and 4 require the slant board to be turned away so that the feet are angled down.

Position 4

Place a strap around your knees and pull out against the strap and release it twenty times. After this initial set of pushouts and releases, push out against the strap and maintain constant pressure on the strap for the following foot/ankle movements.

Using the muscles on the back of your lower leg, push your heels up off the slant board so that only the balls of your feet and toes are in contact with the board. Return your heels to the slant board and repeat twenty times. Keep continuous pressure between your big toe and the slant board as your raise your heel and go up onto your toes. Then, using the muscles on the front side of the lower leg, lift the balls of your feet and toes up off the slant board so only your heels are in contact with the board. Return your toes to the slant board and repeat twenty times.

Static Extension

KNOW IT: Improves pelvic and spine imbalance to improve load joint function.

DO IT: Kneel on a block or ottoman with your hands on the floor. Shift your hips forward six to eight inches so that your hips are slightly in front of your knees. Work your hands out in front of you until your hands are directly under your shoulders. Let your back and head drop toward the floor and your shoulder blades come together. Relax your abs. Try to tilt your butt toward the ceiling and notice the pronounced arch in your lower back.

OWN IT: Hold for one or two minutes.

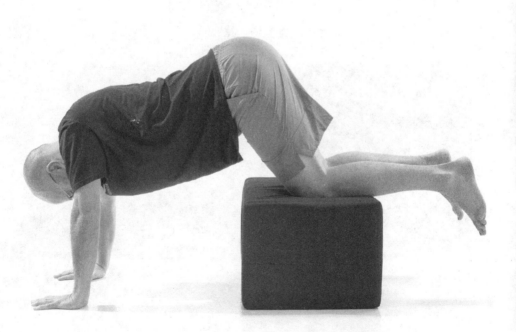

Static Back

KNOW IT: Settles your hips and back, releasing the compensating muscles that interfere with balance and functional movement.

DO IT: Lie on your back with both legs bent at right angles on a chair or block. Your hips should also be at ninety-degree angles. Rest your arms on the floor outstretched at forty-five-degree angles, with your palms up. Let your back settle into the floor, and breathe from your diaphragm (that is, do stomach breathing). Keep your abs relaxed (an easy test is to see if your stomach is rising and falling with each breath).

OWN IT: Hold this position for five minutes.

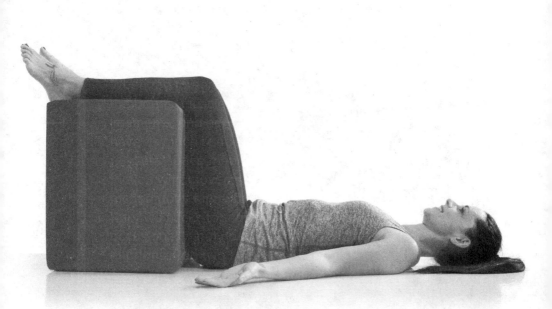

Pullovers

KNOW IT: Improves shoulder mobility and reduces compensation in the thoracic spine.

DO IT: From the Static Back position, clasp your hands together tightly with your fingers interlaced. Extend your elbows straight to the ceiling. Continuing to hold both arms straight, bring them back over your head, either to the floor or as far as they will go without bending. Return to the starting position with your arms extended straight to the ceiling. Relax your abdominal muscles, and don't rush.

OWN IT: Do fifteen times, three sets.

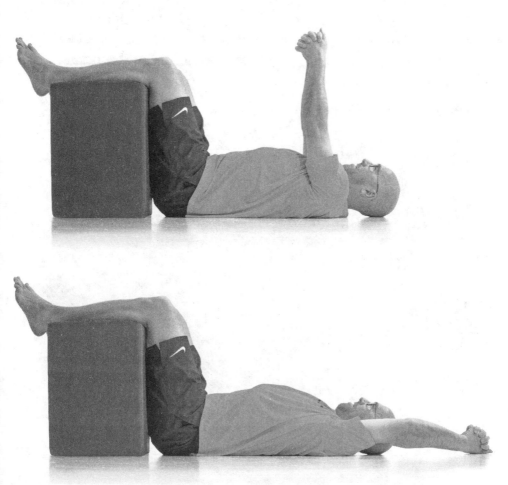

Cats and Dogs

KNOW IT: Works the hips, spine, shoulders, and neck in coordinated flexion-extension.

DO IT: Get down on the floor on your hands and knees. Make sure your knees are aligned with your hips, and your wrists with your shoulders. Your legs should be parallel with each other, and your feet relaxed with your toes pointed. Make sure your weight is distributed evenly. Smoothly round your back upward as your head tucks under to create a curve that runs from your butt to your neck (this is the cat with the arched back). Smoothly sway back down while bringing your head up and arching the back in the opposite direction (this is the gimme-a-treat dog). Try to initiate the movement with your pelvis. Make the two moves flow continuously back and forth rather than keeping them distinct and choppy.

OWN IT: Do one set of ten.

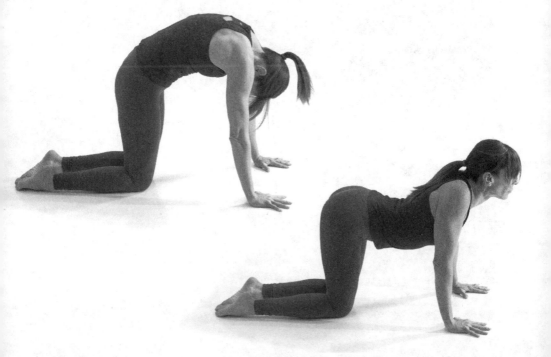

Lucky Number 7

Almost all mammals have the same number of bones in their neck—seven. From mice, to humans, to giraffes, the size of the vertebrae varies but the number does not.

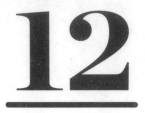

12

Elbows, Wrists, and Hands: Elegant Efficiency

The joints of the upper extremity are true aristocrats. The elbow, wrist, and hand are Jeffersonian joints—elegant, articulate, and refined. They are the means of writing sonnets, reattaching retinas, and flying space shuttles. Capable of light touch or a killing blow, praying or punching, these joints epitomize the ascent of man. And when they hurt, we pay attention.

Much like the knee, the elbow serves as a link between the wrist and the shoulder. The shoulder, being surrounded by larger muscles and directly affected by the torso, can both produce and absorb force on a greater level than the smaller muscles of the forearm and hand. The elbow serves as a transformer, taking the large forces produced at the shoulder and

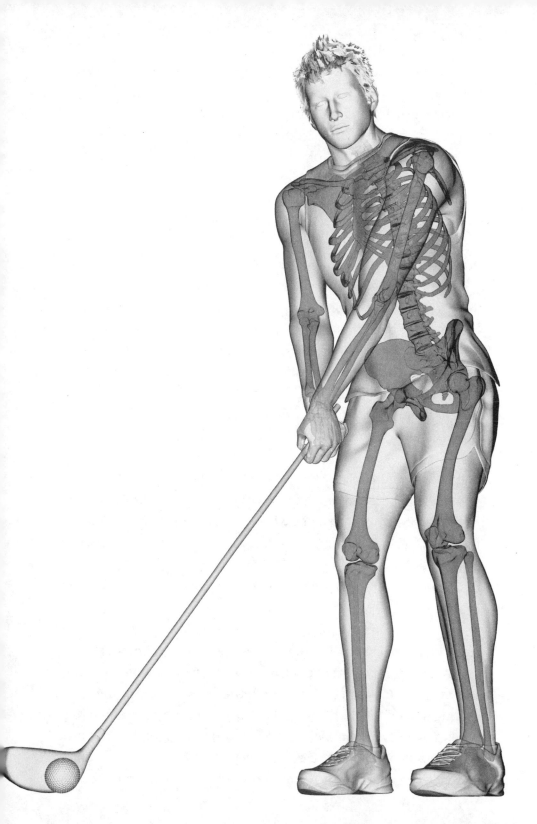

rescaling them to drive the fine, delicate movements of the wrist and hand.

The structure and function of the wrist are like those of the ankle, connecting the two bones of the forearm (the radius and the ulna) with the bones of the hand. Like the ankle, the wrist works with the hand to coordinate our interaction with the environment, establishing a link between the hand and the upper extremity. The combined actions of the hand and wrist allow for fine-tuned, intricate motions while maintaining exquisite and precise control over movement.

The hand is where the mind meets the world. As much as the feet facilitate our unique two-legged gait, the hands enable the use of cognition and intellect that uniquely defines the human species. The ingenuity, imagination, and genius of the human brain are brought to life with our hands. From the early use of tools, to written language, to the development of computer networks and the performance of neurosurgery, the hand connects our cognitive superpowers with our environment.

The hand's sophistication requires years of fine-tuning. A child does not intuitively know how to hold a pencil. Yet with some instruction and practice he will develop the precision necessary to control a pencil while simultaneously developing the cognitive connections necessary for written communication. The development of delicate and exact movement patterns coupled with cognitive skills drive our capacity for exploring and creating.

The function of the hands seems so simple to us, yet the hand is far from simple. Nearly 25 percent of our motor cortex (the area of the brain that controls movement) is devoted to control of the hand. As in the foot, the bones of the hand form three unique arches, which play a critical role in grasping and manipulating objects. These arches are supported and maintained by the muscles of the hand. Disruptions to the balance of the hand muscles can alter the structure of the arches, limiting grip, reduc-

Thumbs Up

Sir Isaac Newton once said, "In the absence of any other proof, the thumb alone would convince me of God's existence." The movement of the thumb seems simple, but its design is complex and its function seemingly flawless. Control of the thumb accounts for 12.5 percent of the motor cortex. That is a lot of command power for a digit that is less than three inches long.

ing the versatility of hand movement, and increasing the amount of stress placed on the surrounding muscles and bones.

The Source Versus the Site of Upper-Extremity Pain

The forearm consists of two bones—the radius and the ulna. Under most circumstances, the upper extremity is intended to rotate as a unit, and these bones lie in parallel to each other. As the shoulder moves, the rest of the arm follows. But we are capable of moving our wrist and hand independent of shoulder motion. To do this, the radius and ulna twist, crossing one on top of the other to allow the hand and wrist to move freely. This advantageous ability makes our upper extremity function all the more versatile. We can reach out from the shoulder and independently move the wrist and hand to accomplish intricate tasks.

When the ball-and-socket function of the shoulder is restricted, the power that comes from the large muscles of the upper arm and torso becomes disconnected from the rest of the arm. No longer connected to move uniformly, the body must exclusively rely on the forearm to power the movements of the hand and wrist.

Much like the added leverage from a wrench makes loosening a bolt much easier, small movements at the shoulder easily power movements of the hand and wrist when the

Forearm Motion

You can picture the movement of the radius and ulna with your index and middle fingers. Hold your hand out, palm down. Your index and middle fingers run in fairly parallel lines with a small, straight space between them. Now cross the middle finger over the top of the index finger. The space between your fingers shrinks and twists. When the forearm rotates, the bones, muscles, tendons, ligaments, and nerves don't have as much space.

Less space means more friction with movement, and friction does funny things. Rub two sticks together occasionally and nothing happens. Rub two sticks together constantly and there's a fire. When our shoulder is misaligned and we rely exclusively on forearm rotation for movement of the wrist and hand, pain is inevitable.

The body's primary weapon against pain is to shut down movement. As the elbow and wrist become stiff, restricted, and painful, movement is slowly diminished. We all instinctively know that this is a last-resort remedy, but in the short run it works. The friction abates and our pain subsides. The elbow and wrist, however, are so central to our modern lives that losing full use of them is a major crisis. As a

musculoskeletal chain is aligned and connected. Those small movements are easy work for the large muscles surrounding the shoulder. But take away the wrench, and suddenly twisting the bolt becomes a much more arduous task. With the shoulder and all its power out of the picture, the muscles of the forearm and hand must work overtime. We can sustain this workload for a time, but without reprieve, the added stress will eventually result in pain and injury.

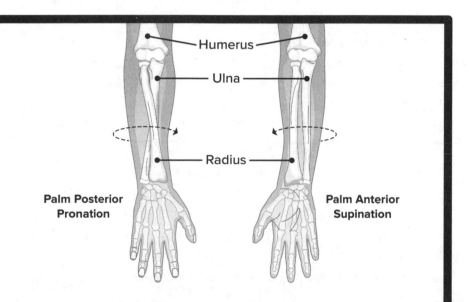

**Palm Posterior
Pronation**

Humerus

Ulna

Radius

**Palm Anterior
Supination**

result, the usual pattern over the long run is a period of relative inactivity to quell the symptoms, followed by a resumption of the demand that caused the friction to begin with. Gradually the relief gained during the periods of inactivity dwindles and the simmering coals of unresolved friction spark

another fire. The only way to extinguish such pain is to realign the joints. When the shoulder and other major load joints are connected and balanced, they freely power the more mundane movements of the upper extremity, freeing our elbows, wrists, and hands to return to their aristocratic ways.

Remote-Control Fingers

We operate our fingers via remote control. Not a single muscle is located within our fingers. Rather, tendons running from muscles located in the hand and forearm connect with the bones of the fingers. Much as guitar strings require tuned tension to produce the desired sound, only tendons with the right amount of tension can optimally perform the task of movement. Too much tension, and the tendons break down from continual shear and strain. Too little tension, and the force generated by the muscles cannot be adequately conducted along the tendons to the fingers.

Many of the muscles that control finger movement originate at the elbow and rely on long tendons to cross the wrist joint and connect with the fingers. Similarly, many of the muscles that control wrist movement originate at the elbow and connect with the wrist and hand via slightly shorter tendons. This is why our forearm is much thicker near the elbow than at the wrist. The thick muscle bodies that power hand and wrist movement sit in the upper forearm with thin connecting tendons running through the lower forearm. This location allows for these muscles to be bigger and stronger than would be possible if they were constrained to the small spaces of the hand and fingers.

Thumb Wars and Small Finger Opposition

The thumbs are critical to the dexterity we have come to take for granted when it comes to hand function. Nine muscles are dedicated to the movement of the thumb. Its function is so important that nature divided the control of those muscles between all three of the nerves that innervate the hand, adding a layer of protection from the potential loss of function with an isolated nerve injury.

Muscleless Fingers!

Not a single muscle is located in our fingers. Rather, we control our finger movement remotely, with long tendons connecting muscle bodies in the hand and forearm with the bones of our fingers.

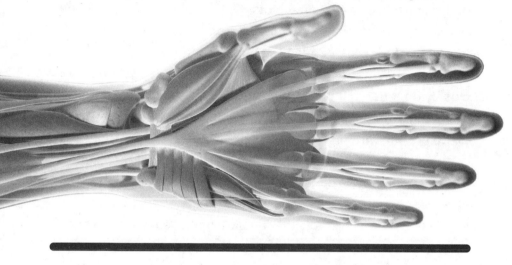

Many people think that possessing opposable thumbs makes humans unique when it comes to hand function. While the ability to position the thumb opposite to the fingers is relatively uncommon in the animal world, it is a trait we share with all primates. What is unique is our ability to rotate our fourth and fifth fingers across the palm to meet our thumb. That trait allows for the unique strength and versatility of the human grip.

Out-of-Balance Injuries

There is a pandemic of overuse injuries in modern society. Tennis elbow, golfer's elbow, shoulder tendinitis, wrist tendinitis—the list of injuries thought to result from repetitive motion is extensive and overwhelming. But here is the thing— our joints were designed to move repetitively. If we can walk around the Earth four times during our life span, with the same repetitive joint movement occurring with each stride, it does not make sense that our joints would have some preprogrammed, finite capacity for movement. Movement is not the problem when it comes to overuse injuries. The problem is balance—or lack thereof. Imbalanced movement creates abnormal stress on the muscles, bones, and joints. Overuse injuries are a result of that abnormal stress. It would be much more correct to call them out-of-balance injuries.

When it comes to staying balanced, the hand and wrist closely depend on the elbow and shoulder. Many of the muscles that control the wrist and hand attach to the humerus (the bone of the upper arm). The humerus runs the entirety of the upper arm, connecting with the shoulder joint. When the shoulders slump forward, the rotation of the humerus changes. Because the muscles that control the wrist and hand are attached to the humerus, persistent rotation disrupts the function of these muscles. That imbalance changes the dynamics of hand and wrist movement, and since we use our hands all day, every day, that imbalance inevitably catches up with us. The abnormal strain created by repetitive improper movement fuels pain in the forearm and hand, but the imbalance that needs to be fixed starts two feet higher.

Carpal Arch

Carpal tunnel is arguably the most famous upper-extremity overuse injury. But guess what? It too can be more readily explained as an out-of-balance injury. Overuse becomes relevant only when something is out of balance and causing abnormal irritation and strain. With carpal tunnel, that something is one of the hand's arches. The median nerve runs through a channel of bones that form at the base of the hand. That channel is small, and the median nerve shares it with seven tendons running from muscles in the forearm to the hand and fingers. When the shape of that bony channel changes, the nerve and the surrounding tendons are compressed into a smaller space. Nerves

The Carpal Tunnel

The median nerve runs through the carpal tunnel. Muscle imbalance and dysfunction change the size of the carpal tunnel and predispose the nerve to irritation.

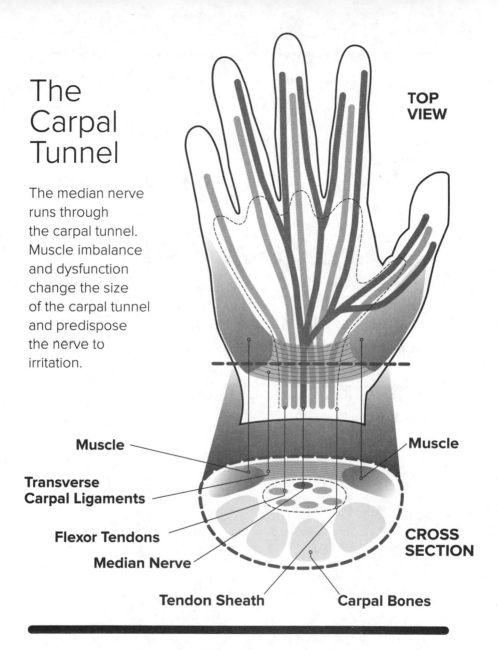

TOP VIEW

Muscle

Muscle

Transverse Carpal Ligaments

Flexor Tendons

Median Nerve

CROSS SECTION

Tendon Sheath

Carpal Bones

do not like to be compressed. Neither do tendons. Nerve compression results in tingling, numbness, and weakness in the hand. Tendon compression results in irritation and swelling, further restricting the space inside the carpal tunnel. The cure is to restore the balance of the hand muscles, re-creating the arch at the base of the hand and giving the nerve room to breathe.

The Menu for Elbows

Standing Chest Openers,
Unilateral...251

Standing Chest Openers,
Bilateral..252

Hanging..253

Wall Elbow Curls............................254

Static Extension.............................255

Wall Clock.......................................256

Cats and Dogs................................258

Progressive Supine Groin.............259

Standing Chest Openers, Unilateral

KNOW IT: Improves humerus and scapula range of motion and balances shoulder motion with motion of the thoracic spine.

DO IT: Stand sideways to a wall, an arm's length away from it, with your feet pointed straight and hip-width apart. Extend your inside arm and place your palm flat on the wall with your fingers spread apart. Try to flatten your entire palm against the wall and spread your fingers as far apart as you can. Your outside arm is hanging down at your side. Relax your stomach. Keeping your arm straight, rotate it forward and backward from the shoulder. Do not bend your elbow, and do not raise your shoulders. Do not move your hand. Keep your hand flat against the wall throughout the movement. Now turn so your opposite side is facing the wall and repeat on that side.

OWN IT: Do two sets of ten repetitions on each side.

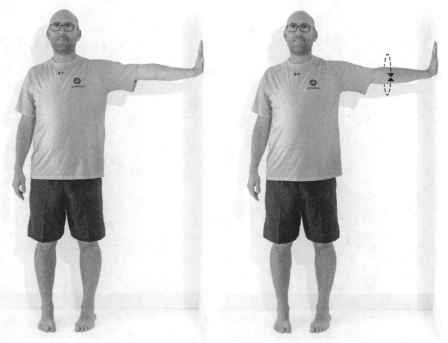

Standing Chest Openers, Bilateral

KNOW IT: Improves scapula and shoulder range of motion and reduces thoracic spine and torso imbalance.

DO IT: Stand facing a wall, an arm's length away from it, with your feet pointed straight, hip-width apart. Place your palms flat on the wall with your fingers spread apart. Keeping your arms straight, rotate your arms in and out from the shoulders. Do not bend your elbows, do not raise your shoulders, and do not move your hands. Your stomach should be relaxed. Try to flatten your entire palm against the wall and spread your fingers as wide as possible. Keep both hands flat against the wall throughout the entire movement.

OWN IT: Do two sets of ten repetitions.

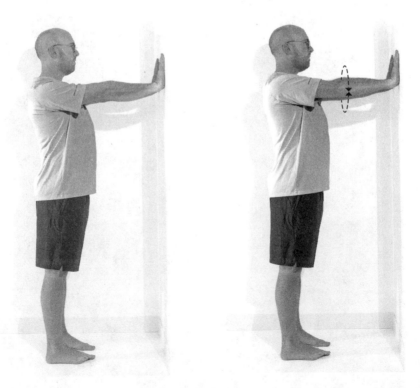

Hanging

KNOW IT: Elongates the muscles along the posterior side of the body, which often become tight and imbalanced from a lifestyle with too much sitting.

DO IT: Stand with your feet hip-width apart and pointed straight ahead. Bend over to touch your toes and hang, allowing the shoulders to relax. Drop your head and try to concentrate on relaxing your upper back. Keep your thighs tight and do not bend your knees or bounce. Keep your hips in line with your knees and ankles (don't stick your butt out behind you). If your hands don't reach the ground, let your arms hang loosely and allow gravity to slowly pull you closer to the ground. If your hands touch the ground, place your palms down with your fingers extended and allow gravity to slowly flatten your hands against the ground.

OWN IT: Hold for one minute.

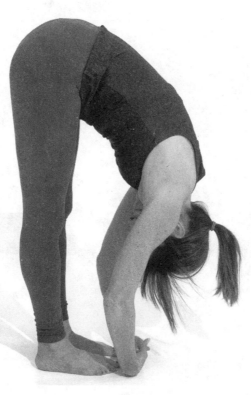

Wall Elbow Curls

KNOW IT: Promotes proper positioning of the load joints and synchronizes scapula movement with thoracic extension and flexion.

DO IT: Stand against a wall with your feet pointed straight ahead. Keep your heels, hips, and upper back against the wall. Your hands should be in golfer's grip, with your fingers curled, knuckles flexed, and thumbs extended. Place your knuckles against your temples with your thumbs pointed down to your shoulders. Keeping your elbows bent, open your elbows and spread them to the side until the backs of your arms contact the wall. Then bring your elbows back together until the inside of your elbows touch. Your elbows should come together directly in front of you, not off to one side or the other.

OWN IT: Do one set of twenty-five repetitions.

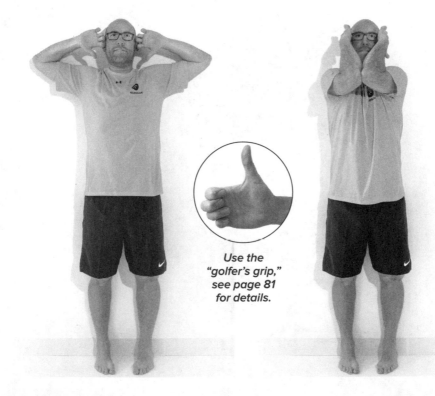

Use the "golfer's grip," see page 81 for details.

Static Extension

KNOW IT: Improves pelvic and spine imbalance to improve load joint function.

DO IT: Kneel on a block or ottoman with your hands on the floor. Shift your hips forward six to eight inches so that your hips are slightly in front of your knees. Work your hands out in front of you until your hands are directly under your shoulders. Let your back and head drop toward the floor and your shoulder blades come together. Relax your abs. Try to tilt your butt toward the ceiling and notice the pronounced arch in your lower back.

OWN IT: Hold for one or two minutes.

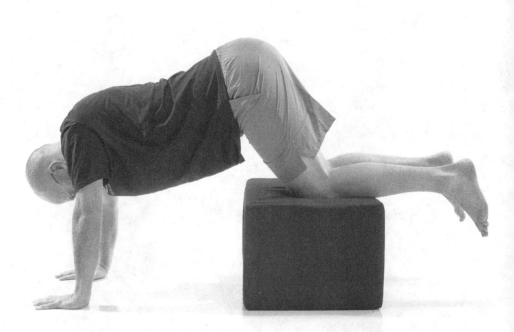

Wall Clock

KNOW IT: Improves function of the scapula. The shoulder blades should move up and down, back and forth, clockwise and counterclockwise. When they don't, much of the dynamic interaction within the torso is lost.

DO IT: If this position aggravates your elbow pain, drop it from the sequence initially and then try again a few days later. When it no longer brings pain, integrate it into your sequences.

1. Face the wall, and place your feet in a pigeon-toed position up against the wall. Place your arms over your head in the 12 o'clock position, and hold for one minute. Your el-

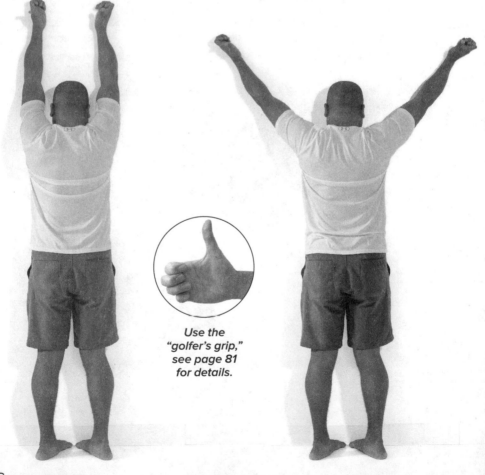

Use the "golfer's grip," see page 81 for details.

bows should be straight, and your hands in golfer's grip with your fingers curled, knuckles flexed, and thumbs extended. Your thumbs should be pointing away from the wall. Rotate your arms away from your body, initiating the movement with your shoulders. Continuously try to increase the external rotation of your arms throughout the exercise. Hold for one minute.

2. Remain in the same pigeon-toed stance. Place your arms over your head in the 10 and 2 position and repeat the previous movement. Keep your arms straight and your hands in golfer's grip with your fingers curled, knuckles flexed, and thumbs extended and pointed away from the wall. Continuously rotate the arms externally from the shoulders. Hold for one minute.

3. Place your arms in the 9 and the 3 position (straight out horizontally) and repeat the previous movement. Keep your arms straight and your hands in golfer's grip with your fingers curled, knuckles flexed, and thumbs extended and pointed away from the wall. Continuously rotate the arms externally from the shoulders. Hold for one minute.

Cats and Dogs

KNOW IT: Works the hips, spine, shoulders, and neck in coordinated flexion-extension.

DO IT: Get down on the floor on your hands and knees. Make sure your knees are aligned with your hips, and your wrists with your shoulders. Your legs should be parallel with each other, and your feet relaxed with your toes pointed. Make sure your weight is distributed evenly. Smoothly round your back upward as your head tucks under to create a curve that runs from your butt to your neck (this is the cat with the arched back). Smoothly sway back down while bringing your head up and arching the back in the opposite direction (this is the gimme-a-treat dog). Try to initiate the movement with your pelvis. Make the two moves flow continuously back and forth rather than keeping them distinct and choppy.

OWN IT: Do one set of ten.

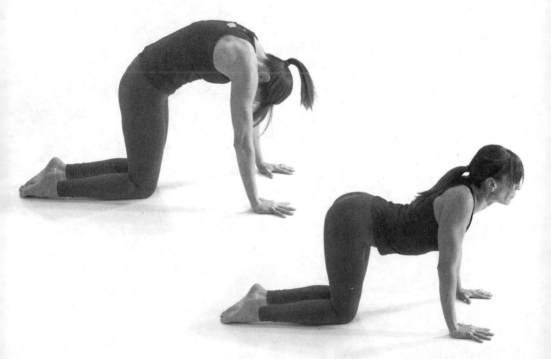

Progressive Supine Groin

KNOW IT: Allows for proper flexion and extension of the leg while reducing compensating side-to-side and rotational motions.

DO IT: Lie on your back with one leg resting on a block or chair, your knee bent at a ninety-degree angle, while the other leg is extended on a small stepladder, a stack of books, or something of a similar height (so that your back and hips are flat on the floor). Prop the outside of your foot on the extended leg to prevent it from rolling out. Let the leg rest at this top level for three to five minutes. Ideally, your lower back should come to rest flat against the floor before moving on. Lower your extended foot about five to eight inches and repeat for three to five minutes. Continue to progressively lower your extended foot five to eight inches at a time until your foot is resting against the floor. Again, let the leg rest along the floor until your lower back rests flat on the floor. Don't try to flatten your back.
Let it happen naturally.

OWN IT: Hold each position for three minutes, and repeat on the opposite side.

These images depict Progressive Supine Groin using the Egoscue tower, a tool specifically designed for the exercise. You can complete the exercise without the tower as described above.

The Menu for Hands/Wrists

Shoulder Shrugs..............................261

Shoulder Rolls 262

Standing Wall with Block..............263

Standing Quad Stretch.................264

Hanging.......................................265

Wall Clock....................................266

Air Bench.....................................268

Shoulder Shrugs

KNOW IT: Promotes proper position of the scapula and thoracic extension, while reducing imbalance in the torso and spine.

DO IT: Stand with your back to a wall, feet pointing straight ahead, against the wall and hip-width apart, arms hanging down at your sides. Your hips and upper back should be against the wall. Squeeze your shoulder blades together and hold them together while you shrug your shoulders up and down. Keeping your shoulder blades together is key. You should hear your upper back and shoulder blades gliding on the wall as the shoulders move up and down. Don't let your shoulders roll forward (keep your shoulder blades pinned back). Relax your abs.

OWN IT: Do two sets of ten repetitions.

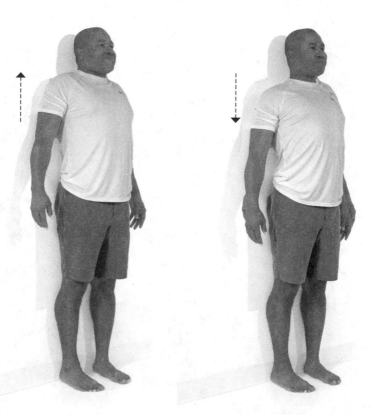

Shoulder Rolls

KNOW IT: Promotes proper position and movement of the scapula and shoulder and reduces imbalance in the torso and spine.

DO IT: Stand with your feet pointing straight ahead and hip-width apart. Your arms are relaxed at your sides. Circle your shoulders by pulling your shoulders back, then up, and then forward, then down. This full sequence is one "roll." Do two sets of ten rolls. Now reverse the circle by pulling your shoulders forward, then up, then back, then down. This full sequence is one "roll." Do two sets of ten rolls.

OWN IT: Do two sets of ten rolls in each direction.

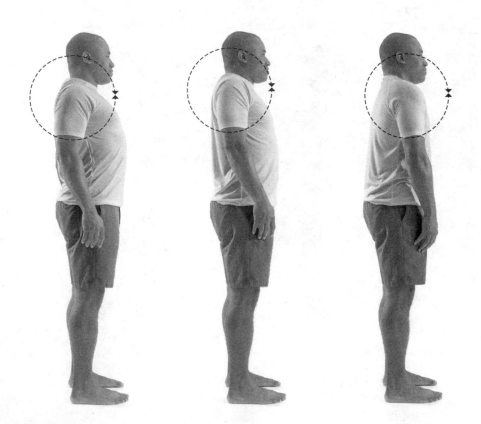

Standing Wall with Block

KNOW IT: Promotes proper positioning of all load joints.

DO IT: Stand at a wall with your heels, hips, and upper back against the wall. Place a small block or pillow between your knees. Apply gentle pressure, just enough to hold the pillow in place; do not push into it. It's okay if your head is not against the wall. Stand in a relaxed position and let your head rest naturally. With enough time, your head will move back on its own; don't force it. Relax your stomach and your arms and allow your body to adjust to this new position. Keep your thighs tight so that your knees are locked in a straight, or extended, position. Remember to keep your feet pointed straight ahead and your stomach relaxed throughout.

OWN IT: Hold for six to eight minutes.

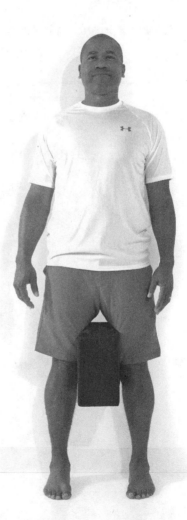

Standing Quad Stretch

KNOW IT: Helps to balance the quadriceps and hamstring muscles to balance pelvis and torso position.

DO IT: Stand on one foot and bend the other leg back, placing the top of the foot on a block or the back of a chair. Let the ankle relax so the foot is pointed. The height will dictate the amount of stretch in the quadriceps. Keep your hips and shoulders square. Tighten the thigh muscle on the straight leg and try to keep your bent knee directly underneath your hip. Tuck your hips under to feel the stretch. If necessary, hold on to something for balance.

OWN IT: Hold for one minute on each side.

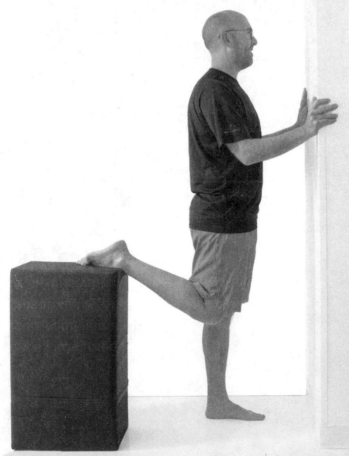

Hanging

KNOW IT: Elongates the muscles along the posterior side of the body, which often become tight and imbalanced from a lifestyle with too much sitting.

DO IT: Stand with your feet hip-width apart and pointed straight ahead. Bend over to touch your toes and hang, allowing the shoulders to relax. Drop your head and try to concentrate on relaxing your upper back. Keep your thighs tight and do not bend your knees or bounce. Keep your hips in line with your knees and ankles (don't stick your butt out behind you). If your hands don't reach the ground, let your arms hang loosely and allow gravity to slowly pull you closer to the ground. If your hands touch the ground, place your palms down with your fingers extended and allow gravity to slowly flatten your hands against the ground.

OWN IT: Hold for one minute.

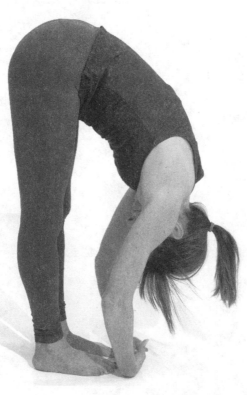

Wall Clock

KNOW IT: Improves function of the scapula. The shoulder blades should move up and down, back and forth, clockwise and counterclockwise. When they don't, much of the dynamic interaction within the torso is lost.

DO IT: If this position aggravates your elbow pain, drop it from the sequence initially and then try again a few days later. When it no longer brings pain, integrate it into your sequences.

1. Face the wall, and place your feet in a pigeon-toed position up against the wall. Place your arms over your head in the 12 o'clock position, and hold for one minute. Your el-

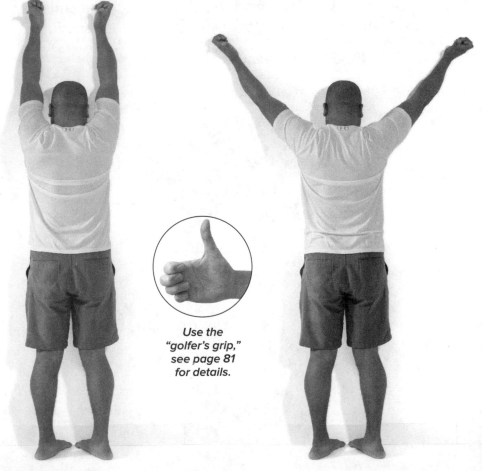

Use the "golfer's grip," see page 81 for details.

bows should be straight, and your hands in golfer's grip with your fingers curled, knuckles flexed, and thumbs extended. Your thumbs should be pointing away from the wall. Rotate your arms away from your body, initiating the movement with your shoulders. Continuously try to increase the external rotation of your arms throughout the exercise. Hold for one minute.

2. Remain in the same pigeon-toed stance. Place your arms over your head in the 10 and 2 position and repeat the previous movement. Keep your arms straight and your hands in golfer's grip with your fingers curled, knuckles flexed, and thumbs extended and pointed away from the wall. Continuously rotate the arms externally from the shoulders. Hold for one minute.

3. Place your arms in the 9 and 3 position (straight out horizontally) and repeat the previous movement. Keep your arms straight and your hands in golfer's grip with your fingers curled, knuckles flexed, and thumbs extended and pointed away from the wall. Continuously rotate the arms externally from the shoulders. Hold for one minute.

Air Bench

KNOW IT: Puts the hips, knees, and ankles simultaneously into flexion while they are under load.

DO IT: Stand with your back to a wall, and press your hips and the small of your back into the wall while walking your feet forward and sliding into a sitting position. Stop just before your hips reach a ninety-degree angle. Your knees should also be close to a ninety-degree angle, but your ankles should be just slightly forward of your knees. **Note:** If you feel pain in your knees, raise your body up the wall to relieve the pressure. Make sure your lower back is pressed against the wall and keep it pressed against the wall throughout the exercise. You should feel your quadriceps working along the top of the thigh.

OWN IT: Hold for one to three minutes. If that is too much, hold for as long as you can and work your way up.

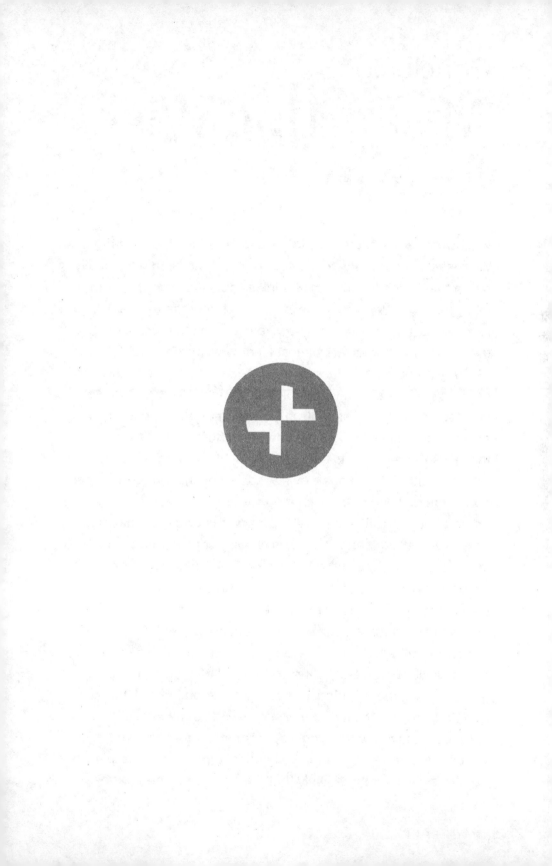

Conclusion:
My Parting Wish for You

We humans are a curious lot. We love to talk about change. We make serious plans to change. And on occasion we actually begin to attempt those plans—think about all the people who join gyms each January. Now think about how the gym looks by the middle of February. The New Year's resolution crew, despite the best of intentions, are almost all nowhere to be found.

Why is change so elusive? My experience has taught me it is not because we are lazy, uninformed, or unmotivated. Change represents the greatest of all challenges, not because it requires effort or discipline. In my experience, we humans have plenty of that. Change represents the greatest of all challenges because it requires faith: Faith in one's own wisdom, instincts, and personal commitment. Faith that the change we are striving to make is going to be a positive change. Faith that the end goal that drove us to make all our serious plans is within our grasp. Faith in our instinct to head right at the fork instead of our usual left despite all the circling thunderheads of uncertainty.

Change is elusive because it requires a leap of faith. It requires trust in yourself. Too often, the changes we seek to make are someone else's idea. The promised outcomes are someone else's wisdom or rule set. Our world is full of well-intended experts—yes, me included. But our experts' beliefs fail if they don't match your reality, your wisdom, and your instinct.

"I don't have the time, energy, or commitment to change." I encourage you to avoid the self-critical tape we tend to play in our heads. It is far more likely that the proposed change does not match your truth than it is that you are actually lazy, unmotivated, or incapable.

My forty-plus years of work have taught me this: No one knows more about you than you do. You are the unequivocal expert on you. I have yet to meet a single person who did not have the wisdom to understand the real cause of their pain. I have never met a single client who didn't instinctively know what to do to solve their pain issues. My purpose in this book has been to talk to your instinct, your wisdom, your truth. My hope is that in doing so you might be willing to take that leap of faith in yourself.

Or better yet—that you already have. Think back to when we started this journey. I asked you a seemingly simple question that would serve as motivation along the path to becoming pain free. What can't you do now that you would like to do?

Now that we have completed our exploration of the functional realities of the human body, my hope is that you are well on your way to returning yourself to a balanced state and a pain-free life. So now I will offer up a new question—one that I hope will ignite a feeling of self-satisfaction and pride but will also continue to motivate you along your journey. What can you do now that you couldn't do before?

If you can answer that, you have a new truth that you didn't possess when we started this journey. Even if it is only a small something, a stepping-stone along the way to where you ultimately want to arrive, you have proven to yourself that you have the power to change your circumstance. You trusted your wisdom, instinct, and truth, and you arrived safely with a positive change. You read this book, you performed the exercises, and now you can do something that you previously could not.

Whether it's big or small, you made that change. The first leap of faith is always the hardest. Now, on to the next. What else can't you do that you would like to do? Keep trusting your truth and the possibilities are endless.

Acknowledgments

This book is my seventh, thanks to the perseverance of my friend and literary agent Margret McBride. Margret started our literary journey in 1982 when she walked into my office with a big smile and a "you have something to say."

A book project is a very difficult task for me, because I am not a detailed and focused author. This means it is necessary to assemble a team of professionals who have the skills necessary to get the project to print. This team must have the patience and energy to make sense of my thought process—not an easy feat!

This trip was made easier by Ted Spiker, who provided a reasoned and calm perspective on the text. George Karabotsos provided similar perspective and design expertise for the look, layout, and illustrations throughout the book. My editor, Elana Seplow-Jolley, was patient, involved, and easy to work with, a rarity in my experience with editors. And finally, thanks to Faye Atchison, Margret's right-hand woman and a fan of my work, for all the tireless, behind-the-scenes effort that went into making this book a reality.

Thanks to my longtime associate and friend Brian Bradley, whose energy for this project kept my eye on the ball. Thanks to my Egoscue family for continuously inspiring and motivating me. These dedicated therapists have made me proud every day of the last four decades, helping countless individuals become pain free. And a special thanks to John Lynch for his kind words in the foreword and his willingness to publicly share his Egoscue journey.

The heaviest lifting on this book was done by Meta Haley, MD, who worked long hours wordsmithing my thoughts. She took my form of disjointed communication, translated it into a comprehendible message, and ultimately composed this understandable text. This book would not have happened without her.

To my readers, thank you for your continued support and encouragement. Your success and health are the most important and energizing part of my work.

And finally, to my late wife, Troi; thank you for your tireless, and eventually successful, effort to convince me that the best was yet to come.

Notes

14–15 **Astronauts can lose up to 20 percent** Brooks, N. "Five Things That Happen to Your Body in Space." *Phys.org.* (January 18, 2016). https://phys .org/news/2016-01-body-space.html.

20 **Movement also increases the production of dopamine** Basso, J. C., Suzuki, W. A. "The Effects of Acute Exercise on Mood, Cognition, Neurophysiology, and Neurochemical Pathways: A Review." *Brain Plasticity* (Amsterdam, Netherlands) 2(2) (March 28, 2017): 127–152. doi:10.3233 /BPL-160040.

22 **The average person checks their phone** "You Will Spend 76,500 Hours, or Almost 9 Years of Your Life, Using Your Mobile Device." *Entrepreneur* (November 24, 2020). https://www.entrepreneur.com/article/360320.

32 **MRIs of the brain following immobilization** Langer, N., Hänggi, J., Müller, N. A., Simmen, H.P., Jäncke, L. "Effects of Limb Immobilization on Brain Plasticity." *Neurology* 78(3) (January 17, 2012): 182–188. doi: 10.1212 /WNL.0b013 e31823fcd9c. PMID: 22249495.

38 **Ed Whitlock ran the Toronto Marathon** Longman, J. "85-Year-Old Marathoner Is So Fast That Even Scientists Marvel." *The New York Times* (December 29, 2016). https://www.nytimes.com/2016/12/28/sports/ed -whitlock-marathon-running.html.

40 **80 percent of adults** "Osteoarthritis." Cleveland Clinic. Accessed June 29, 2021. https://my.clevelandclinic.org/health/diseases/5599-osteoarthritis.

40 **MRI findings in the lower back** Brinjikji, W., Luetmer, P. H., Comstock, B., et al. "Systematic Literature Review of Imaging Features of Spinal Degeneration in Asymptomatic Populations." *American Journal of Neuroradiology* 36(4) (2015): 811–816. doi:10.3174/ajnr.A4173.

41 **MRIs performed during acute episodes** Hashmi, J. A., et al. "Shape Shifting Pain: Chronification of Back Pain Shifts Brain Representation from Nociceptive to Emotional Circuits." *Brain: A Journal of Neurology* 136(9) (2013): 2751–68. doi:10.1093/brain/awt211.

66 **Approximately one in every ten people** Kadakia, A. R. "Our Knowledge of Orthopaedics. Your Best Health." *OrthoInfo* (June 2010). https://ortho info.aaos.org/en/diseases-conditions/plantar-fascitis-and-bone-spurs.

94 **increases the strength of our quadriceps** Fox, A. J., Wanivenhaus, F., Rodeo, S. A. "The Basic Science of the Patella: Structure, Composition, and Function." *Journal of Knee Surgery* 25(2) (May 2012): 127–41.

127 **average American sits for 10 hours a day** "Get America Standing. Active and Productive Working. Sit-stand Solutions." Accessed September 29, 2020. https://getamericastanding.org/.

128 **Almost 70 percent of people who undergo hip** Cawley, D. T., Guerin, S. J., Walsh, J., Simpkin, A., Masterson, E. L. "The Significance of Hand Dominance in Hip Osteoarthritis." *Semin Arthritis Rheum* 44(5) (April 2015): 527–530. doi: 10.1016/j.semarthrit.2014.11.001. Epub (Nov. 12, 2014): PMID: 25498323.

165 **Dehydration can limit this critical function** Zhu, Q., Gao, X., Brown, M. D., Temple, H. T., Gu, W. "Simulation of Water Content Distributions in Degenerated Human Intervertebral Discs." *Journal of Orthopaedic Research* 35(1) (2016): 147–53. https://doi.org/10.1002/jor.23284.

213 **hornlike spikes on the back of the skull** Shahar, D., Sayers, M. G. L. "Prominent Exostosis Projecting from the Occipital Squama More Substantial and Prevalent in Young Adult Than Older Age Groups. *Scientific Reports* 8 (2018): 3354. https://doi.org/10.1038/s41598-018-21625-1.

215 **head weights in photograph** Hansraj, K. K. "Assessment of Stresses in the Cervical Spine Caused by Posture and Position of the Head." *Surgical Technology International* 25(25) (2014): 277–279.

216 **Vision is our most powerful sense** Sells, S. B., Fixott, R. S. "Evaluation of Research on Effects of Visual Training on Visual Functions." *American Journal of Ophthalmology* 44(2) (August 1957): 230–236.

218 **Individuals with decreased or reversed** Bulut, M. D., et al. "Decreased Vertebral Artery Hemodynamics in Patients with Loss of Cervical Lordosis." *Medical Science Monitor: International Medical Journal of Experimental and Clinical Research* 22 (February 15, 2016): 495–500. doi:10.12659/msm .897500.

218 **dramatic improvement in the rate** Katz, E. A., et al. "Increase in Cerebral Blood Flow Indicated by Increased Cerebral Arterial Area and Pixel Intensity on Brain Magnetic Resonance Angiogram Following Correction of Cervical Lordosis." *Brain Circulation* 5(1) (2019): 19–26. doi:10.4103/bc .bc_25_18.

220 **small changes in cervical spine position** Fanton, M., Kuo, C., Sganga, J., Hernandez, F., Camarillo, D. "Dependency of Head Impact Rotation on Head-Neck Positioning and Soft Tissue Forces." *IEEE Transactions on Biomedical Engineering* 66(4) (2019): 988–999. https://doi.org/10.1109 /tbme.2018.2866147.

242 **Nearly 25 percent** "Motor Cortex" (Section 3, Chapter 3). Neuroscience Online: An Electronic Textbook for the Neurosciences: Department of Neurobiology and Anatomy—The University of Texas Medical School at Houston." Accessed September 29, 2021. https://nba.uth.tmc.edu /neuroscience/m/s3/chapter03.html.

243 **12.5 percent of the motor cortex** Dubuc, B. "The Motor Cortex—The Brain from Top to Bottom." Canadian Institutes of Health Research: Institute of Neurosciences, Mental Health, and Addiction. Accessed August 12, 2020. https://thebrain.mcgill.ca/flash/d/d_06/d_06_cr/d_06 _cr_mou/d_06_cr_mou.html.

Index

abdominal muscles, 17, 34, 121, 164

Abduction-Adduction with Narrow and Wide Feet, 83

acetabulum, 122, 123

Achilles tendon, 64, 66–68

ACL (anterior cruciate ligament), 101

Active Wishbone, 138

adaptation, 30–32

age, pain and, 38–40

Air Bench
    in back menu, 171, 174
    in feet menu, 78
    in hand and wrist menu, 268
    in head and neck menu, 227
    in hip and pelvis menu, 151
    in knee menu, 119
    in shoulder menu, 202

ambulation, 58

ankle, see feet and ankle

annulus fibrosus, 161

arches, 58–59, 61, 62, 65

arthritis, 39–40
    in hips, 128
    in knees, 97, 128

articular cartilage, 96

astronauts, 14–16

back, 101, 121
    E-cises for, 166–81
    muscle spasms, 162
    muscles, 156–58, 162, 188
    pain, 5–7, 34, 41, 51, 61
    scoliosis, 159
    see also spine

balance, 18, 19, 26, 27, 45–46, 48, 52, 54, 55, 58, 60, 64, 68, 126, 128, 160, 163, 164, 216, 217, 248

ball-and-socket joints, 122, 125, 184, 185, 243
blood flow, 218–20
bones, 16, 18, 19, 26, 32, 36
Bradley, Brian, 7
brain, 20, 32–33, 41, 42, 210, 216, 218, 219, 242
bulging discs, 160
bunions, 63

calcaneus (heel bone), 57, 59, 64, 66
Calf/Hamstring Stretch, 76
calf muscles, 62, 65, 67–68
Campbell, John, 29
cannabinoids, 20
cardiovascular system, 36
carpal tunnel, 248–49
cartilage, 97–100, 128
Cats and Dogs, 41
    in ankle menu, 85
    in elbow menu, 258
    in headache menu, 238
    in hip and pelvis menu, 144, 150
    in knee menu, 105, 109, 115, 118
    in shoulder menu, 201, 209
cell phones, 22, 212
cerebrospinal fluid, 19
cervical (neck) spine, 153–56, 158, 210–11, 218–20
childbirth, 129
children, 5, 13–14, 214
coccyx, 155
compensation, 30–32, 34, 156, 188
concussions, 219, 220
contracting muscles, 156, 164
Cook, John, 21
cramps, leg, 69
Cross-Crawling, 87
CT scans, 6, 39

dehydration, 69, 165
depression, 20
digestion, 19

Dillberg, Dustin, 23

dizziness, 216–17

dopamine, 20

dorsiflexion, 61

downward gaze, 212, 213

drug addiction, 20

dynamic tension, law of, 16, 18

Eastern medicine, 23

E-cises (Egoscue Method), 7, 15, 21, 33, 41, 43, 45–54

    Abduction-Adduction with Narrow and Wide Feet, 83

    Active Wishbone, 138

    Air Bench, *see* Air Bench

    in ankle menu, 79–89

    in back menu, 166–81

    Calf/Hamstring Stretch, 76

    Cats and Dogs, *see* Cats and Dogs

    Cross-Crawling, 87

    in elbow menu, 250–59

    in feet menu, 70–78, 230–34

    Flexion Knee Pillow Squeezes, 103

    Floor Block, *see* Floor Block

    Foot Circles and Point Flexes, 75, 88–89, 136

    Frog, 74

    Gravity Drop, 140

    in hand and wrist menu, 260–68

    Hanging, *see* Hanging

    in head and neck menu, 221–27

    in headache menu, 228–38

    Hero's Pose, 225

    Hip Lift, 134

    in hip menu, 131–51

    Hooklying Rocking Chair, 133, 146

    in knee menu, 102–19

    Kneeling Counter Stretch, 139

    Lying Supine, *see* Lying Supine

    Modified Floor Block, *see* Modified Floor Block

    Pelvic Tilts, 135, 148

    in pelvis menu, 131–51

    Progressive Supine Groin, *see* Progressive Supine Groin

    Pullovers, *see* Pullovers

E-cises (Egoscue Method) (*cont'd*):
    Reverse Presses, 177
    Seated Arm Circles, 207
    Short Foot, *see* Short Foot
    in shoulder menu, 193–209, 261, 262
    Shoulder Rolls, 262
    Shoulder Shrugs, 261
    Sitting Floor, 206
    Sitting Heel Raises with Block, *see* Sitting Heel Raises with Block
    Sitting Knee Pillow Squeezes, *see* Sitting Knee Pillow Squeezes
    Slant Board Ankle Sequence, 230–34
    Squat, *see* Squat
    Standing Arm Circles, 80
    Standing Chest Openers, Bilateral, 252
    Standing Chest Openers, Unilateral, 251
    Standing Forward Bend, 108
    Standing Wall with Block, *see* Standing Wall with Block
    Static Back, *see* Static Back
    Static Back with Knee Pillow Squeezes, *see* Static Back with Knee
        Pillow Squeezes
    Static Extension, *see* Static Extension
    Static Wall, 84
    Three-Position Toe Raises, 197
    Unilateral Supine Femur Rotations, 147
    Wall Clock, *see* Wall Clock
    Wall Elbow Curls, 254
    Wall Stork, *see* Wall Stork
Egoscue tower, 111, 200, 259
Einstein, Albert, 45
elbows, 7, 240–49
    E-cises for, 250–59
    joints, 240
    overuse injuries, 247
electrolyte imbalance, 69
emotional volatility, 41
endorphins, 20
exercise, *see* E-cises (Egoscue Method)
external stimuli, 26

fascia, 61
fatigue, 41, 42

feet
    muscles, 60–62, 65, 68–69
feet and ankles, 16, 17, 56–69, 90, 96
    Achilles tendon, 64, 66–68
    arches, 58–59, 61, 62, 65
    bones, 57, 58, 63, 68–69
    bunions, 63
    E-cises for, 70–89, 136, 230–34
    flat feet, 61
    heel spurs, 66
    leg cramps, 69
    plantar fasciitis, 61, 64–66
    shin splints, 68–69
    shoes, 58, 65, 66
    sprains, 61
femoral head, 123
femur, 67, 68, 91, 93, 96–99, 101, 122–25, 185
fibula, 57, 59, 64, 91, 93, 101
fingers, 246–47
fixed flexion, 157
flat feet, 61
flexion-extension of knees, 92
Flexion Knee Pillow Squeezes, 103
Floor Block
    in back menu, 179
    in hip and pelvis menu, 137
Foot Circles and Point Flexes, 75, 88–89, 136
forward head position, 212, 213, 215, 216, 218
fragility, pain as sign of, 40–42
Frog, 74

gastrocnemius, 67
glenoid socket, 185
gluteal muscles, 121
Golfer's Grip, 80, 81, 137, 254, 266
gorillas, 154, 155
gravity, 14–16, 156, 158, 164, 212, 213, 217
Gravity Drop, 140
growth spurts, 214

hamstring muscles, 17, 121

hand and wrist, 51, 182, 240–49
  bones, 242, 243, 249
  carpal tunnel, 248–49
  E-cises for, 260–68
  fingers, 246–47
  function of, 242
  joints, 240
  muscles, 242, 249
  overuse injuries, 247, 248
  thumbs, 243, 246–47

Hanging, 143
  in elbow menu, 253
  in hand and wrist menu, 265

head and neck, 159–60, 183, 188, 210–20
  bones, 211, 239
  cervical spine and, 210–11
  concussions, 219, 220
  E-cises for, 221–27
  forward head position, 212, 213, 215, 216, 218
  headaches, see headaches
  joints, 211, 212
  muscles, 211, 212, 214, 215, 218
  pillows and, 218–19

headaches, 217–18
  E-cises for, 228–38

heart, 19, 158

heel spurs, 66

Heiden, Eric, 33

herniated discs, 5–6, 47, 160–62
  E-cises for, 166–74

Hero's Pose, 225

Hip Lift, 134

hip replacements, 128, 130

hips, 7, 15–17, 90, 101, 120–30, 184
  arthritis in, 128
  childbirth and, 129
  E-cises for, 131–51
  flexion and extension of, 124–28
  joints, 122, 185

muscles, 123, 126–27, 188
    upper and lower body triangles, 190–91
Hodgson, Paul, 7
Hooklying Rocking Chair, 133, 146
hopelessness, 42
hormones, 20
hornlike spikes, 213
humerus bone, 183, 184, 185, 189, 245, 248
hunchback, 163
hydration, 165
hypersensitivity, 41

internal stimuli, 26, 28
intervertebral disc, 161, 214
intestines, 19
intravertebral disc, 160, 162, 165
isolation, 20, 22

joint braces, 101
joint effusion, 98
joints, 16–18, 26, 32, 36, 38
    ankle, 57, 59–60
    ball-and-socket, 122, 125, 184, 185, 243
    cartilage, 97–100, 128
    feet, 57, 58, 63, 65, 68–69
    hand and wrist, 240, 242, 243, 249
    head and neck, 211, 212, 239
    hips, 122, 185
    knee, 91, 92, 97, 98
    leg, 91, 101
    pelvis, 123–24
    sacroiliac, 123
    shoulder, 183–85, 188, 189, 245

kidneys, 36, 158
kinesthetic sense (muscle memory), 13, 22, 46, 48
Kneeling Counter Stretch, 139
knees, 16, 17, 40, 90–119
    ACL (anterior cruciate ligament), 101
    arthritis in, 97, 128

knees (*cont'd*):
    E-cises for, 102–19
    flexion-extension, 92
    joints, 91, 92, 97, 98
    meniscus, 98, 99
    muscles, 92, 94–95
    patella (kneecap), 93, 94, 97
    signs of problems, 96–97

Lahav, Loren, 39
Lardon, Michael, 33
lateral meniscus, 93
leg cramps, 69
ligaments, 93, 98, 101, 123
liver, 158
loneliness, 20
lower-body triangles, 190–91
lower limb pain, 61
lumbar curve, 157
lumbar (lower back) spine, 152–58, 211
    E-cises for, 166–74
lungs, 19, 36, 158, 163, 218
Lying Supine
    in back menu, 173
    in knee menu, 116
Lynch, John, 21

medial meniscus, 93
median nerve, 248–49
medications, 3, 34, 345
meniscus, 98, 99
metabolic rate, 19
metatarsal joint, 63
Miller, Jack, 43
Modified Floor Block
    in back menu, 169
    in knee menu, 117
molecules, 20
motion, *see* E-cises (Egoscue Method)
motor cortex, 242

motor units, 38–39

MRI (magnetic resonance imaging), 5–7, 32, 38–41

muscle atrophy, 20, 29, 156, 164

muscle spasms, 162

muscles, 16–20, 26, 29–34, 36, 38–42
    back, 156–58, 162, 188
    calf, 62, 65, 67–68
    feet, 60–62, 65, 68–69
    hand and wrist, 242, 249
    head and neck, 211, 212, 214, 215, 218
    hips, 123, 126–27, 188
    knee, 92, 94–95
    pelvis, 121, 126–27
    shoulder, 184, 188–90
    spine, 155–60, 162–64
    thumb, 246

myokines, 20

neck, see head and neck

neurotransmitters, 20

Newton, Sir Isaac, 243

Nicklaus, Jack, 33

nucleus pulposus, 161

orthotics, 66

osteoarthritis, 39–40

overpronation, 58

overuse injuries, 247–48

oxygen, lack of, 218–20

pain
    as adaptive consequence, 26–32
    age and, 38–40
    cycle of, 8–11
    fear of, 4–5, 8–9, 14
    as messenger, 35–36
    as sign of fragility, 40–42
    understanding, 35–44

painkillers, 345

patella (kneecap), 93, 94, 97

patience, 42

Pelvic Tilts, 135, 148
pelvis, 15, 18, 101, 120–30, 154, 184, 185
    childbirth and, 129
    connection with upper and lower body, 124–28
    E-cises for, 131–51
    hip flexion and extension and, 124–28
    importance of, 120–22
    joints, 123–24
    muscles, 121, 126–27
    sitting and, 126–27
peristalsis, 19
pillows, 218–19
plantar fasciitis, 61, 64–66
plantarflexion, 61
posture, 21, 23, 50–52, 127
Progressive Supine Groin
    in elbow menu, 259
    in knee menu, 110–11
    in shoulder menu, 200
pronation, 58, 59
proprioception, 216
proteins, 20
psoas muscles, 34, 121
Pullovers
    in back menu, 178
    in headache menu, 237

quadriceps muscle, 17, 94, 121

radius, 242–45
reaching up, 188
Reed, Simon, 47
respiratory muscles, 163
Reverse Presses, 177
risk aversion, 22
rotator cuff, 159, 184, 188–90

S-curve of spine, 18, 152, 154–56, 163, 164, 213, 218
sacroiliac joints, 123
sacrum, 155

Sandison, Heather, 15

scapula, 183, 184, 185, 189

scoliosis, 159

Seated Arm Circles, 207

sedentary lifestyle, 10, 14, 20, 22–23, 95, 126–27, 188, 213, 214

self-reliance, 5, 9, 11, 50

self-test, 52, 53

Shea, Steven, 51

shin splints, 68–69

shock absorption, 58, 62, 165

shoes, 58, 65, 66

Short Foot
   in feet and ankle menu, 72
   in head and neck menu, 223
   in hip and pelvis menu, 142

Shoulder Rolls, 262

Shoulder Shrugs, 261

shoulders, 7, 16, 17, 101, 122, 159–60, 182–209, 248
   bones, 183–85
   E-cises for, 193–209, 261, 262
   joints, 184, 185, 188, 189, 245
   muscles, 184, 188–90
   rotator cuff, 159, 184, 188–90
   upper and lower body triangles, 190–91

sitting, 10, 126–27, 188, 213, 214

Sitting Floor, 206

Sitting Heel Raises with Block
   in feet and ankle menu, 71, 82
   in shoulder menu, 196

Sitting Knee Pillow Squeezes
   in back menu, 167
   in head and neck menu, 226
   in shoulder menu, 195, 204

skull, 93, 122, 213

Slant Board Ankle Sequence, 230–34

sleep, 165

slipped discs, 160

space voyages, 14–16

spinal fusions, 162

spine, 15–18, 93, 122, 152–65
    cervical, 153–56, 158, 210–11, 218–20
    E-cises for, 166–81
    herniated discs, 5–6, 47, 160–62, 166–74
    lumbar (lower back), 152–58, 211
    muscles, 155–60, 162–64
    S-curve of, 18, 152, 154–56, 163, 164, 213, 218
    sitting and, 126–27
    surgery, 160, 162
    thoracic (upper back), 153–56, 158–60, 163, 211
Squat
    in back menu, 181
    in shoulder menu, 208
Standing Arm Circles, 80
Standing Chest Openers, Bilateral, 252
Standing Chest Openers, Unilateral, 251
Standing Forward Bend, 108
Standing Quad Stretch
    in hand and wrist menu, 264
    in knees menu, 107
Standing Wall with Block
    in hand and wrist menu, 263
    in head and neck menu, 222
    in headache menu, 229
    in knee menu, 113
    in shoulder menu, 194–95
Static Back
    in back menu, 172, 176
    in feet and ankle menu, 73
    in head and neck menu, 236
    in hip and pelvis menu, 145
    in knee menu, 104
    in shoulder menu, 199
Static Back with Knee Pillow Squeezes
    in back menu, 168
    in hip and pelvis menu, 132
Static Extension
    in back menu, 170, 180
    in elbow menu, 255
    in feet and ankle menu, 77, 86
    in head and neck menu, 180, 224, 235

in hip and pelvis menu, 149
in knee menu, 106
in shoulder menu, 205
Static Wall, 84
stimulus, 26, 28, 31, 41
suicide, 20
supination, 58, 59
surgery, 5
hip replacements, 128, 130
spine, 160, 162
synovial fluid, 98, 100

talus (ankle bone), 57, 59, 64
technology, 5, 6, 10, 11, 22, 25, 28
tendinitis, 247
thoracic (upper back) spine, 153–56, 158–60, 163, 211
Three-Position Toe Raises, 197
thumbs, 243, 246–47
tibia, 57, 59, 64, 68, 91, 93, 96–99, 101
traumatic brain injury, 219
two-legged ambulation, 18

ulna, 242–45
uncertainty, 43–44
Unilateral Supine Femur Rotations, 147
upper-body triangles, 190–91

vertebrae, 152, 158, 160, 162
vertical loading, 16–18
vestibular input, 216
video games, 50–52
vision, 216
visual input, 216

waist-hip ratio, 129
Wall Clock
in elbow menu, 256–57
in hand and wrist menu, 266–67
Wall Elbow Curls, 254

Wall Stork
    in knee menu, 114
    in shoulder menu, 198
water consumption, 165
Weis, Laurie-Ann, 49
Whitlock, Ed, 38–39
wrist, *see* hand and wrist

X-rays, 6, 38, 39, 66

zero gravity environment, 15

About the Author

Pete Egoscue is a former Marine and the founder of The Egoscue Method. Over the last forty-plus years, he has enabled millions of people to lead pain-free lives. His exercise therapy programs are acclaimed worldwide for treating musculoskeletal pain attributed to workplace and sports injuries, accidents, aging, and other conditions. He has consulted with some of the biggest names in sports, business, and politics. He has previously published six books, focused on empowering everyone, regardless of their walk in life, to take control of their health and journey to a pain-free, movement-filled life.

Egoscue is the chairman and CEO of Egoscue, Inc. and operates thirty-plus clinics in the United States, Mexico, and Japan. He lives in Park City, Utah.